NECK AND
ARM PAIN

NECK AND ARM PAIN

Edition 2

RENE CAILLIET, M.D.

Professor and Chairman
Department of Rehabilitative Medicine
University of Southern California
School of Medicine
Los Angeles, California

F. A. DAVIS COMPANY • Philadelphia

Also by Rene Cailliet:

FOOT AND ANKLE PAIN
HAND PAIN AND IMPAIRMENT
KNEE PAIN AND DISABILITY
LOW BACK PAIN
SCOLIOSIS
SHOULDER PAIN
SOFT TISSUE PAIN AND DISABILITY
THE SHOULDER IN HEMIPLEGIA

Copyright © 1981 by F. A. Davis Company

Second printing 1981
Third printing 1982

Printed in the United States of America

**Library of Congress Cataloging in Publication
Data**

Cailliet, Rene.
  Neck and arm pain.

  Includes bibliographical references and
index.
  1. Neck pain. 2. Brachialgia. I. Title.
[DNLM: 1. Arm. 2. Neck. 3. Pain.
4. Shoulder.   WE805   C134n]
RC936.C26   1981   617'.53   80-17352
ISBN 0-8036-1609-0

Preface to Second Edition

Over the years since the first edition of *Neck and Arm Pain* there have been numerous additions and changes in diagnostic procedures and in treatment concepts of these syndromes. The second edition is presented in an attempt to update these newer concepts.

Cervical myelopathy was omitted from the previous edition and neglected a very important consideration of painful, disabling aspects of cervical spine disease. The frequency of cervical spondylosis causing myelopathy yet being unrecognized encouraged me to add this important chapter to the second edition.

Numerous concepts of treatment, both surgical and nonsurgical, always benefit from careful review and revision. Numerous theories of local pain and referred pain are always being reviewed clinically and in research laboratories and their pertinence to clinical application needs to be reviewed for the busy clinician who has too little time to assimilate and make applicable these many factions of a common clinical syndrome.

The medical-legal aspect of painful and disabling conditions is continually mandating better medical evaluation and patient care. A better educated patient population also expects better informed medical care delivery as well as explanation of a painful, disabling condition.

The following statement by a legal specialist in a medical journal well summarizes these thoughts:

> Cervical trauma is one of those areas of physical injury which like head and back injuries, often results in subjective complaints that are extremely difficult for the courts, industrial commissioners, insurance carriers and attorneys to properly evaluate. Leading neurosurgical and orthopedic specialists tell us that there is still much that is unknown about the pathology of cervical trauma, that many times they do not know exactly what to look for in injuries

to this area, and that they usually cannot deny subjective complaints in view of lack of precise information.*

This revision has been prepared in an attempt to add to this knowledge. It is always with the idea that specialists will also benefit but, more importantly, that students, interns, residents of all specialties, and practitioners of every field of medicine will acquire a sufficient knowledgeable basis for evaluation and treatment of the patient suffering from cervical spine pathology. This is the purpose of the second edition of *Neck and Arm Pain*.

RENE CAILLIET, M.D.

---

*Allen, W. S.: Medical-legal aspects of cervical trauma. Clin. Neurosurg. 2:106–13, 1954.

Preface to First Edition

Of all the musculo-skeletal and neuromuscular conditions causing pain and disability in man, pain and dysfunction originating in the neck, shoulders, and upper extremities is exceeded only by low back pain.

The early manifestations of neck pain and the significance of limited motion are frequently overlooked because of ignorance of normal functions and abnormal deviations. In later life, neck pain and its sequelae are attributed to *aging* or to the *wear and tear of life*. Sufferers from these effects would have benefitted from earlier recognition and a more physiological approach to treatment.

The musculo-skeletal system must be fully understood in its *static* anatomical sense and in its *kinetic* function before abnormality and the mechanism of pain production and dysfunction can be recognized and understood. Pathological changes can be prevented; and when a complete reversal of abnormal changes is impossible, at least the symptoms and disability caused by these changes can be ameliorated.

The neck in this monograph is discussed in a didactic, positive manner principally from the author's viewpoint. The bibliography is small and selective regarding the more controversial aspects, but the text is based on voluminous literature as well as personal observation and opinion.

The *stick-man* drawings and the simplified sketches have been effective in similar monographs and as teaching aids in the classroom. They are used here to aid the busy practitioner, the burdened medical student or intern, and the practicing physical therapist; and they should be helpful as well in informing the patient during office practice.

I owe my publishers a debt of gratitude for offering this text in an inexpensive paperback volume. This manner of presenting medical texts brings medical information in a practical, low-cost form to the physician who is staggered by the annual deluge of medical texts.

I am sincerely grateful to the physicians of the *Gaylord Seminar* under the direction of Sidney Licht, M.D., who reviewed the manuscript and made invaluable constructive criticisms.

RENE CAILLIET, M.D.

Contents

Illustrations xi
Introduction xv

Chapter 1. Functional Anatomy 1
  Anterior Portion of the Functional Unit 1
  Posterior Portion of the Functional Unit 7
  Static Spine 8
  Posture 9
  Kinetic Spine 11
  Ligamentous Support 18
  Musculature of the Neck 21
  Tissue Sites of Pain Production 23
  The Cervical Nerves 27
  The Sympathetic Nervous System 34
  Upper Cervical Segments 38

Chapter 2. Neck Pain Originating in the Soft Tissues 42

Chapter 3. Diagnosis of Neck Pain 50
  Physical Examination 51
  X-Ray Examination 52

Chapter 4. Cervical Disk Disease as a Factor in Pain and
Disability 56
  Nature and Mechanism of Radicular Pain 56
  Cervical Disk 62
  Localization of Root Level by Clinical Examination 64

Chapter 5. Subluxations of the Cervical Spine Including the
"Whiplash" Syndrome 73

Syndrome of Acute Central Spinal Cord Injury 90
Diagnosis of Deceleration Sprain Injury 92

Chapter 6. Degenerative Disk Disease **94**

Chapter 7. Cervical Spondylotic Myelopathy **106**
Symptoms 111
Prognosis 112
Examination 112
Laboratory Findings 112
Myelography 113
Treatment 115

Chapter 8. Treatment: General and Specific **118**

Chapter 9. Differential Diagnosis **137**
Anterior Scalene Syndrome 139
Claviculocostal Syndrome 143
Pectoralis Minor Syndrome (Hyperabduction Syndrome) .. 145
Scapulocostal Syndrome 145
Fibromyositis 146
Pericapsulitis Shoulder Pain 150
Shoulder-Hand Syndrome 154
Carpal Tunnel Syndrome 154
Brachial Plexus Neuritis (Plexitis) 156

Index **159**

Illustrations

1. The functional unit 2
2. Hydraulic mechanism of the intervertebral disk 3
3. Elasticity of annulus fibers 4
4. Comparative lateral views of cervical and lumbar
    functional units 5
5. Comparative curves of cervical and lumbar spine:
    Related to disk shapes 5
6. Vertebral bodies of cervical and lumbar region:
    Comparing joints and disks 6
7. Static spine considered erect posture 8
8. Chronological development of cervical lordosis 10
9. Gravity effect on a "forward head" posture with
    increased lordosis 12
10. Composite movements of the cervical spine 13
11. Occipital-atlas movement 13
12. Rotation of the atlas about the odontoid process of the
    axis 14
13. Locking mechanism of C_2 on C_3 15
14. "Gliding" movement in flexing spine 15
15. Alteration in spinal canal length 16
16. Foraminal closure in head lateral flexion and turning ... 17
17. Influence of sequence upon neck flexion 19
18. Ligamentous support of the neck 20
19. Translatory gliding on cervical flexion 21
20. Musculature of the head and neck 22
21. Sites of major muscle bulk in the cervical spine 23
22. Tissue sites of pain production 24
23. Postulated mechanism of "disk pain" (sciatica or
    brachialgia) 25

24. Pain production from myofascial-periosteal strain and muscle ischemia 27
25. Component fibers of a cervical nerve 28
26. Formation and location of cervical nerve roots 29
27. Nerve root location with regard to disk level 30
28. Direction of foraminal grooves 30
29. Reaction of the dura in neck flexion and extension 31
30. Relationship of nerve root within foramen during neck movement 32
31. Anatomical boundaries of the intervertebral canal 33
32. Dura-arachnoid sleeve of nerve root in the intervertebral canal 35
33. Cross section of contents of intervertebral canal 36
34. Periradicular sheath of nerve 37
35. Sympathetic nervous system of the cervical region 38
36. Vertebral artery pathway 39
37. Upper cervical functional units 40
38. Reflex mechanism for relief of cramps: Concept 45
39. Mechanisms by which irritations result in functional disability 46
40. Unilateral subluxation from excessive rotation 47
41. Referral sites of pain elicited by intranuclear diskogram . 58
42. Movement of nerve roots about their point of attachment 60
43. Comparison of lumbar and cervical disk containers 63
44. Possible results from direction of disk herniation 65
45. Muscle examination of the triceps (C_7) 66
46. Muscle testing—external rotators (C_5) 67
47. Brachioradialis reflex 68
48. Pronator reflex 69
49. Sixth cervical nerve root irritation 70
50. Seventh cervical nerve root irritation 70
51. Eighth cervical nerve root irritation 71
52. Hyperextension injury 75
53. Muscle spindle system 76
54. Muscular reaction to "whiplash" injury 77
55. Mechanism of hyperflexion sprain injury to the neck 78
56. Tissues involved in hyperflexion sprain injury of the neck 79
57. Hyperextension-hyperflexion injury 79
58. Rear-end impact with neck hyperextension sprain 80
59. Flexion phase of acceleration injury to the neck (sprain) . 81
60. Compression theory of "whiplash" injury 82
61. Compression-plus-torque theory of cervical injury resulting from "whiplash" 83

62. Mechanism of disk injury 83
63. Effect of deceleration injury to neck with head turned .. 85
64. Sites of fracture-dislocations in the cervical spine 87
65. Dermatomal areas of occipital nerves 88
66. Referral areas of upper cervical roots 89
67. Vascular supply to the cervical cord 91
68. Evolutionary stages of disk degeneration 95
69. Mechanism of spondylosis 96
70. Disk degeneration with formation of "spondylosis" 97
71. Sagittal diameter of the cervical spinal canal 98
72. Normal nutrition and lubrication of posterior articulation 99
73. Mechanism of osteoarthritic changes in facet joints 100
74. Foraminal opening variations 101
75. Sites of greatest osteophyte formation 102
76. Effect of posture upon cervical spine 103
77. Gravity effect upon cervical lordosis 104
78. Sensory and motor tracts of the spinal cord 108
79. Spinal cord arterial supply 109
80. Spinal arterial supply 109
81. Spinal canal stenosis: Neck extension 110
82. Spinal canal stenosis: Neck flexion 111
83. Spinal canal width 112
84. Measurement of subluxation 113
85. Measurement of cervical spine flexion-extension 114
86. Soft cervical collar 120
87. Cervical collar: Pattern for construction 121
88. SOMI cervical orthosis 122
89. Cervical pillow 123
90. Bed cervical traction, hospital type 126
91. Supine traction 127
92. Overhead cervical traction for home use 127
93. Angle of traction on head halter 128
94. Home cervical traction—not recommended 129
95. Recording of range of motion 130
96. Localization of painful segment 131
97. Rhythmic stabilization exercises to neck 133
98. Posture training—distraction 134
99. Brachial plexus (schematic) 138
100. Supraclavicular space 139
101. Scalene anticus syndrome 141
102. Scapular elevation exercise—seated 142
103. Scapular elevation exercises—standing 143
104. Claviculocostal syndrome and pectoralis minor
       syndrome 144

105. Scapulocostal syndrome 146
106. Trigger zones 150
107. Glenohumeral movement 151
108. Scapulohumeral rhythm of shoulder movement 153
109. Carpal tunnel syndrome 155

Introduction

The patient complaining of neck, head, shoulder, or arm pain presents the examiner with a condition that must be anatomically localized, mechanically understood, and pathologically classified. The site of pain specified by the patient may be the source of pain, or it may merely be the area to which the pain is referred. The tissues involved in producing the pain must be identified, and the manner in which they are irritated to cause the pain must be understood. The pathological changes resulting from the irritated tissues must be ascertained as removable, reducible, or irreversible. In order to treat the pain syndrome, all these factors must be known so that the maximum relief of symptoms, the greatest degree of reversal of the pathology, and the utmost in prevention of progression or recurrence is obtained.

Interpretation of neck, shoulder, and arm pain applies the axiom *if characteristic pain can be reproduced by a position or a movement and the exact nature of that position or movement is understood, the mechanism of pain production is also understood.*

The patient describes the type, location, character, frequency, and duration of the pain, as well as its relationship to position or movement. After careful questioning the patient associates certain neck movements with precipitating or relieving the pain. Statements such as, "I painted a ceiling," or, "I worked for a long time in a cramped position under my car," imply a position of the neck or upper back that preceded the onset of symptoms.

The history of pain felt only when "looking up" or "turning the head to the left" or "reaching behind my back with my arm in dressing," all signify movements and use of the head or arm that lead to the pain. These movements point to the mechanism of pain production. Relief by a change of position must also be analyzed to ascertain "what is happening anatomically and functionally" that is decreasing the painful irritation to the tissues. The physical examination of the patient determines the anatomical and tissue sites, and the mechanism by which the symptoms are produced; and it suggests the pathological changes that may be causing or influencing the pain. A careful history is paramount in reaching a diagnosis; a careful examination is necessary to verify the diagnosis. As in most clinically painful conditions, X-rays and laboratory tests are necessary to the diagnosis but per se are of limited significance.

The cervical spine, the thoracic outlet region (so-called cervical-dorsal outlet), and the upper extremities are composed of numerous soft tissues: muscles, ligaments, capsules around joints, and the joints themselves with their cartilage linings and lubricating fluid. Most of these tissues are well supplied with pain nerve endings. All these tissues are compacted into small areas and are subjected to numerous movements, stresses, and strains.

It has been stated that the major causes of neck, shoulder, and arm pain are *arthritis* and *trauma*. These may be the principal conditions leading to discomfort and disability, but they are vague, broad terms needing clarification. It would probably be more correct to state that pain in and from the neck results from the mechanical factor of *encroachment of space* and *impairment of movement*.

Decrease in the space in which pain-sensitive tissues lie or through which they pass compresses these tissues, resulting in possible pain and loss of function. Pain is more apt to occur if pressure is acute and transient, whereas loss of function is more likely if pressure is prolonged and continuous. The sites at which tissues are most likely to be compressed are the intervertebral foramina and within the spinal canal. The tissues in these specific areas are nerves and their coverings, blood vessels, ligaments, joint capsules, and dura matter. Encroachment of space resulting in pressure upon these tissues may result in pain or loss of function.

Impairment of movement of any part of the cervical spine can be responsible for pain, discomfort, and disability. Movement of the neck requires that the disks be of sufficient integrity to allow distortion and recovery, that the ligaments have adequate laxity to permit motion, and that the posterior joints be sufficiently separated, with capsular elasticity and smooth articular surfaces, to permit movement in all directions necessary for normal neck movement. Impairment of movement at any of these points—the disks, ligaments, or joints—may result in limitation, which in itself may be painful and may ultimatedly result in an encroachment of space by causing mechanical irritation, disrupting normal relationships within the functional units, and causing repair factors to invade the foramina. Injury, stress, and faulty mechanics of the neck are capable of irritating the soft tissues of the neck responsible for flexibility.

Steindler* states that the two most frequent causes of cervical pain are *arthritis* and *trauma*. Both are interrelated in their mechanism of producing pain and disability, because they both cause encroachment of space and impairment of motion. Trauma causes pain and impaired function by affecting the soft tissues of the neck and the ultimate effect on motion and space resulting from these soft tissue changes. "Arthritis" implies an inflammatory reaction of joints to injury, stress, or infection. In the neck, "arthritis" is more often a condition of *repair* against stress and injury than a condition caused by infection.

The definition of the term *spondylosis* currently used synonymously with the term *osteoarthritis* is not generally accepted. Spondylosis is most often used to describe degenerative changes of a vertebral joint related to and resulting from diskogenic disease. These degenerative changes are associated with *osteophytosis. Osteoarthritis* may or may not be considered related. It is evident that the term *arthritis* of the cervical spine is used loosely, and it should be clarified in its pathological anatomy and its role of symptom production.

The term "cervical syndrome" has become synonymous with symptoms and signs attributable to irritation of the cervical nerve roots within the region of the cervical intervertebral foramina.† Cervical syndrome applies mostly, if not exclusively, to *cervical radiculitis*. This concept excludes the possibility of pain originating in and from other soft tissues within the neck region where the majority of painful neck syndromes originate and where treatment must be directed to achieve the maximum benefit.

Accurate evaluation of the causes of pain in the neck, shoulder, and arm regions demands knowledge of *functional anatomy.* If the physician does not understand the normal static and kinetic cervical spine, he cannot discern abnormal deviations nor understand the mechanism of pain production. In the absence of understanding functional anatomy the history tells no story and the examination is meaningless. Treatment based on unfounded concepts is bound to fail.

---

*Steindler, A.: The cervical pain syndrome. In: Instructional Course Lectures, The American Academy of Orthopedic Surgeons, vol. 14. Ann Arbor, J. W. Edwards, 1957.
†Jackson, R.: The Cervical Syndrome, ed. 2. Springfield, Ill., Charles C Thomas, 1958.

Functional Anatomy

The cervical spine allows positions and movements that adapt it well to support and move the head. The extent, direction, and variation of movement of this portion of the spine have the greatest range of the entire spinal column. The cervical spine is both a structural, *static* support and a mobile, *kinetic* mechanism.

The cervical spine is an aggregate of superimposed *functional units:* seven vertebrae form the cervical lordotic portion of the vertebral column with each two adjacent vertebrae and their interposed tissues forming a functional unit.

In the lumbar region all *functional units* are basically similar, but the cervical spine has two functional units unique and totally dissimilar from the others: the upper two segments, the occipito-atlanto (skull and first cervical vertebra) and the atlanto-axial unit (C_1–C_2). The remainder of the neck is formed by similar functional units. The units below the axis (C_2), as the lumbar units, consist of an anterior weight-bearing, shock-absorbing portion and a posterior guiding-gliding section (Fig. 1).

ANTERIOR PORTION OF THE FUNCTIONAL UNIT

The anterior portion of the functional unit comprises two vertebral bodies separated by a hydraulic shock-absorbing system called the intervertebral disk (see Fig. 1). The disk is a self-contained fluid elastic system that absorbs shock, permits transient compression, and allows fluid displacement within its elastic container, thus permitting movement and distortion of the functional unit. In this way the major movement of the entire cervical spine occurs (Fig. 2).

The upper and lower plates of the disk are the end plates of the vertebral bodies. These plates are articular hyaline cartilage in direct contact with and adherent to the underlying resilient bone of the

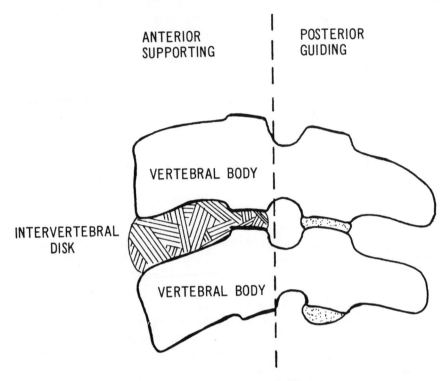

ANTERIOR
SUPPORTING

POSTERIOR
GUIDING

VERTEBRAL BODY

INTERVERTEBRAL
DISK

VERTEBRAL BODY

FIGURE 1. The functional unit in cross section.

vertebral bodies. These inflexible surfaces form the cephalad and caudal walls of the disk.

The outer wall of the disk, the *annulus*, is an interwined fibroelastic mesh that encapsulates the gelatinous matrix of the disk. The annulus fibers are attached around the entire circumference of both upper and lower vertebral end plates and intertwine in crisscross oblique directions. The manner in which these fibers interlace permits movement of one vertebra upon the other in a "rocker" motion, a rotatory direction, and in a horizontal translatory motion (Fig. 3).

The matrix, the *nucleus pulposus*, is contained within the fibrous resilient wall of the annulus and between a floor and ceiling formed by the end plates of the vertebrae. The "elasticity" of the intervertebral disk is attributable to the annulus, not to the fluid content of the nucleus. The nuclear fluid is held within a closed container; thus it conforms to the laws of fluids under pressure. The gel of the *nucleus*, a liquid, cannot be compressed; so any external force exerted upon an area unit is transmitted undiminished to every unit area of the interior of the containing vessel (Law of Blaise Pascal, 1623–1662). The fluid

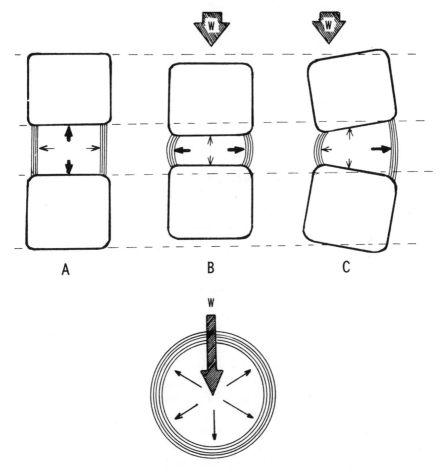

FIGURE 2. Hydraulic mechanism of the intervertebral disk. *A*, Normal disk at rest. Internal pressure exerted in all directions; annulus fibers are taut. *B*, Compressed disk. Fluid of nucleus cannot compress, so annulus must bulge. *C*, Flexion of spine. Fluid shifts; cubic content remains the same; anterior annulus shortens, posterior fibers elongate. *W*, Pressure of gravity of compressive force.

creates an intradiskal pressure that forces the vertebrae apart and keeps the annulus fibers taut. Movement in any direction is permitted by some of the fibers relaxing while the rest remain taut, thus maintaining intradiskal pressure.

The young or undamaged disk has predominantly elastic fibroelastic tissue. Aging and injury to the disk causes larger, less elastic fibers to replace the young, highly elastic collagen fibers. The "older" disk container is thus less elastic.

3

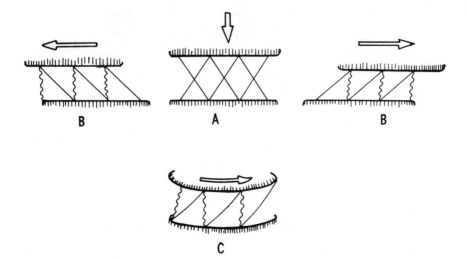

FIGURE 3. Elasticity of annulus fibers. A, Resting functional unit; all fibers taut. B, Lateral shearing (gliding) movements tighten half of fibers, thus maintaining internal tension; half of fibers lose tautness, thus permitting movement. C, Rotation, permitted by same mechanism as lateral shearing.

The colloidal gel of the nucleus pulposus is a mucopolysaccharide that functions by its physical-chemical action; it can imbibe external fluids and maintain its intrinsic water balance. The young disk that contains 80 percent water dehydrates with age and trauma, causing a decrease in the protein polysaccharide and thus a loss in the imbibitory property of the gel. With the loss of intradiskal fluid and the decrease of annular elasticity, a decrease in pressure results.

The intervertebral disk has a vascular supply that disappears after the second decade.[1] By the third decade, the disk is virtually avascular and receives its nutrition by diffusion of lymph through the vertebral end plates. The colloidal imbibitory properties of the gel maintain the disk nutrition. Alternating compression and relaxation of the elastic container, like a sponge being squeezed and released, is a mechanical factor that brings lymph *to* and diffusion *into* the disk. Elasticity of the disk annulus thus is vital to its own nutrition as well as necessary for functional flexibility of the entire spinal column.

Neck motion is limited by the ligaments that connect the vertebrae of the functional units. Excessive movement that would injure the annulus is prevented by the reinforcing ligaments. The ligaments, on the other hand, are sufficiently flexible to allow more translatory gliding motion than is permitted elsewhere in the vertebral column.

The anterior portion of the cervical functional unit has several structural differences from the anterior portion of the lumbar unit. These differences influence the mechanism of movement, the stability of the segment, and the potential functional impairment that can result from injury; but they will be discussed only insofar as they clarify the functional anatomy of the cervical spine.

The vertebral end plates of the lumbar spine are flat and parallel. The nucleus is centrally located in the disk. In the cervical spine, the vertebral cartilaginous plates are concave-convex, and the nucleus is located in the anterior portion of the disk (Figs. 4 and 5). The relation-

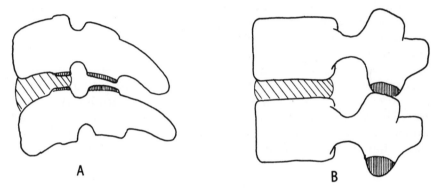

A   B

FIGURE 4.   Comparative lateral views of cervical and lumbar functional units. A, Cervical spine: five joints; disk, paired intervertebral arthroses, and posterior articulations. B, Lumbar spine: three joints; disk, and paired posterior articulations.

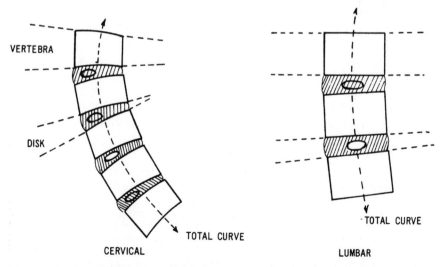

FIGURE 5.   Comparative curves of cervical and lumbar spine: related to disk shapes.

ship of the end plates and their shapes plus the location of the nucleus permits a "rocker" movement between the vertebrae in the lumbar region and a forward and backward "gliding" motion of adjacent vertebrae in the cervical region.[2]

The vertical height of the lumbar disk is only slightly greater anteriorly than posteriorly; thus the upper and lower borders are essentially parallel. In the cervical spine the anterior vertical height of the disk is two times greater than the posterior height, so the disk viewed from the side is wedge shaped. The shape of these disks increases the total curvature of the cervical spine[3] (see Fig. 5).

In the lumbar region, the anterior portion of the functional unit is one of three "joints" of the unit. In the cervical spine three "joints" are located in the anterior portion: five joints in the total functional unit. The two additional "joints" contained in the anterior portion of the cervical functional unit are located along the posterior lateral margin of the vertebral end plate[4] (Figs. 4 and 6). These articular projections are called by various names: uncovertebral joints, intervertebral articulations, lateral interbody joints, or the joints of von Luschka.[4] Although called "joints" they are bony projections that articulate on each other and form false joints, or pseudoarthroses. They are impor-

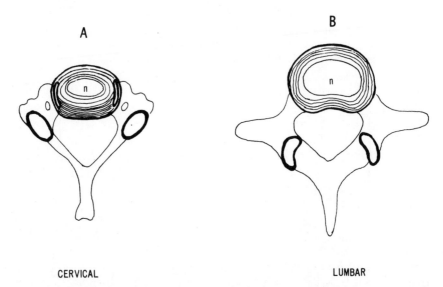

A   B

CERVICAL   LUMBAR

FIGURE 6. Vertebral bodies of cervical and lumbar region: comparing joints and disks. A, Cervical segment. Five joints (including intervertebral articulations). Cervical disks: anterior height 2–3 times greater than posterior. Nucleus, anterior position. Annulus, thicker posterior. B, Lumbar segment. Three joints. Lumbar disks: anterior height slightly greater than posterior. Nucleus, middle position. Annulus, symmetrical.

6

tant in the function of the cervical spine and in the pathology of neck pain and cervical radiculitis. They will be discussed at greater length later.

The annulus in the lumbar region is of symmetrical thickness around the periphery of the disk. The posterior portion of the cervical disk is markedly thicker and broader than the remainder of the annulus (see Fig. 6). This thickened annulus reinforces the disk at vital sites and protects adjacent nerves, blood vessels, and the spinal cord.

The posterior longitudinal ligament of the lumbar spine converges to a point in the caudal area; thus it is incomplete posteriorly in the region of L_3, L_4, L_5, and S_1, inadequately reinforcing the lumbar disk. In the cervical spine, the posterior longitudinal ligament is thick and broad. It is complete across the posterior vertebral area, and between the vertebrae it is actually double layered. This powerful reinforcement is a strong deterrent to disk herniation or bulging, causing major peripheral nerve and spinal cord damage, as will be evident in later chapters.

POSTERIOR PORTION OF THE FUNCTIONAL UNIT

The posterior portion of the functional unit is composed of two vertebral arches, two transverse processes, a central posterior spinous process, and paired articulations. The transverse processes and the posterior spinous process are bony sites of attachment of the neck muscles that move the spine and support the neck and head. Also attached to these bony processes are supporting ligaments.

The posterior articulations, "facets," are true joints. They are synovially lined and are lubricated by synovial fluid within the joint capsule. They are termed apophyseal or zygapophyseal[5] in the sense of being an "outgrowth," but their articular cartilaginous surfaces classify them as true joints, thus capable of degenerative changes referred to as "osteoarthritic" joint changes. The "joints" of von Luschka in the anterior portion of the functional unit do not contain articular cartilage or synovial fluid; therefore they must be considered pseudoarthroses, capable of wear-and-tear degenerative changes but not true osteoarthritic changes.[6]

The posterior facets are in opposition and so placed in direction and degree of inclination as to permit and *guide* the movement of the two adjacent vertebrae. The paired facets are similar in shape and plane from the third cervical vertebra to the seventh cervical vertebra and permit similar movement between these paired joints. The articulations between the skull and the atlas (C_1) and between the atlas (C_1) and the axis (C_2) are unique and require separate description.

7

STATIC SPINE

The cervical spine has a lordotic curve with its convexity anteriorly. The neck curve is balanced in a line with the center of gravity above the dorsal kyphotic curve, in turn superincumbent upon a lordotic curve of the lumbar spine. The primary curve, the lumbar lordosis, upon which all above superimposed curves are dependent, is in turn dependent upon the angulation of the sacral base (Fig. 7). All spinal curves must transect a plumb line to remain in balance with gravity, so an increase of any one curve must be compensated by a proportionate symmetrical increase or decrease in the other two curves. The thoracic

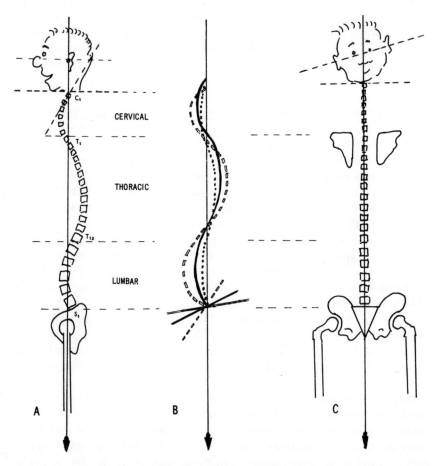

FIGURE 7. Static spine considered erect *posture* (relationship of physiological curves to plumb line of gravity). *A*, Lateral view of erect posture. *B*, Change of superincumbent curves influenced by change of sacral angle. *C*, Anterior-posterior plumb line view with head tilted slightly to one side.

curve varies very little in the anterior-posterior sagittal plane, so any significant alteration of the curvatures must occur in the low back (lumbar lordosis) and in the cervical (lordotic) curves. The clinical significance of the interdependence of the curves is evident when an alteration of the cervical curvature is attempted without considering the total static spinal alignment.

A plumb line center of gravity passes from the external meatus of the ear, transects the odontoid process of the axis (C_1), and transects the bodies of T_1 and T_{12}. It passes through the sacral promontory, slightly posterior to the center of the hip joint, descends anterior to the center of the knee joint, and through the calcaneo-cuboid joint slightly anterior to the lateral malleolus.

A similar plumb line gravity relationship exists when the spinal column is viewed from the front or the back. The plumb line transects the central portion of the vertebral bodies down to the tip of the sacrum midway between both hip joints and both ankles (see Fig. 7). As the lateral view changes with the sacral base angle, so does the anterior-posterior alignment change when the pelvic base deviates from horizontal. If a leg is short, the pelvis drops on that side, and the spine takes off from a tilted pelvis. The plumb line of gravity will influence the spinal curve here, too.

The neck viewed laterally usually forms a symmetrical curve (lordosis) from C_1 to and including C_7. Above C_1 (atlas) there is a sharp angulation[2] to allow the head to be on a level horizontal plane. The cervical spine above C_5, however, may be linear rather than the usual smooth symmetrical curve and be normal, but this is uncommon.

When viewed from the front, the head is usually held slightly tilted to one side.[7] This normal, slight lateral flexion of the head with the rest of the spinal column in the erect position results because the articulations of the atlas and the axis are not in full opposition nor totally symmetrical.

The static, erect spine from the side view showing the four physiological curves depicts, in essence, *posture*.

POSTURE

The spine of the newborn infant has none of the adult physiological curves. The newborn infant remains in the *in utero* posture of total flexion, a curve that is slightly more arched than the ultimate adult kyphosis. No lordotic curves exist in either the cervical or lumbar regions (Fig. 8).

The first lordotic curve begins in the first six to eight weeks of life when the child extends his neck from the prone position and by this antigravity maneuver initiates the muscular action that forms the cer-

9

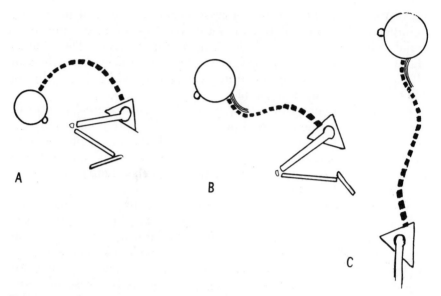

FIGURE 8. Chronological development of cervical lordosis in the development of posture. A, The curve of the fetal spine *in utero*. B, Formation of the cervical lordosis when the head overcomes gravity. C, Erect adult posture.

vical lordosis. The cervical lordosis remains throughout the remainder of the evolution of upright erect position which is man's antigravity destiny. The degree of curve of the neck remains in part influenced by the degree of the other two curves.

Three major factors influence adult posture once the fully erect stance has been reached: (1) inheritance, (2) disease, and (3) habit. Posture is influenced by the familial-hereditary factors in which the posture of the parents and grandparents are carried on to the offspring. This is exemplified in the severe dorsal kyphotic posture, the specific body types, and the short "bull neck." Structural abnormalities influencing posture may be congenital as well as hereditary, or they may result from such disease states as Marie-Strumpell spondylitis or Parkinsonism, to mention a couple. The third influence upon posture, the more insidious and difficult to influence, is the effect of the emotions, habit, and training. Posture to a large degree is a somatic depiction of the emotions. We stand, sit, and move *as we feel*, consciously or unconsciously depicting our attitude of ourselves, our fellow man, and our environment. Posture is "organ language," an outward manifestation of our inner feelings. The fatigued, dejected person will sit or stand with rounded upper back and drooping shoulders. The head will be supported by an excessively arched neck, and held anterior to

10

the center of gravity in a straining, eccentric position. This posture both depicts and causes fatigue, and the strain upon ligaments and demand upon the musculature results in pain.

The tense, hyperkinetic person, by failing to relax, fails to release the tension within his muscles; thus he sustains isometric contractions of his muscles which act as a "vise action" upon the functional units of the neck. Tension, whether emotional or physical—from prolonged tedious activity—affects more often the neck than any other part of the neuro-musculoskeletal parts of the body. "Tension myalgia" of the neck is common, painful, and disabling.

Habit and training affect posture. The tall child who towers over his companions and from self-consciousness or being chided tries to "be smaller" by slumping acquires a round-shouldered posture, inevitably resulting in an increased arching of the neck. The young girl with an unusually large bust may assume a slumped posture to decrease the apparent bust size; thus she molds a posture that may persist throughout her adult life. Without extremely persistent effort to change, the posture assumed in childhood may become structurally fixed.

All postures considered "poor" or undesirable are those aggravating the dorsal kyphosis with a rounding of the shoulders. This faulty posture thrusts the head forward and increases the cervical lordosis. The increase in cervical curve, the position of hyperextension, is the major factor in painful and disabling conditions, as will be seen in the following chapters. Posture, the "static" spine, cannot be overemphasized in its clinical significance[8] (Fig. 9).

KINETIC SPINE

The neck permits movements that adapt it well to its function of supporting the head and allowing the functioning of the sense organs enclosed within the head. Total movement of the neck is the composite of all segmental movements (Fig. 10). All segments move synchronously, but the direction and degree of movement vary at different levels of the segmental spine. The major movement, in both range and amplitude, occurs in the upper portion between the skull and the third cervical vertebra. The major portion of flexion, extension, lateral movement, and rotation occurs between the skull and the atlas and between the atlas and the axis. Below the axis, the extent of movement is dependent upon ligamentous laxity and the distortion and compressibility of the intervertebral disks.

The atlas functions principally with the occiput, and the seventh cervical vertebra (C_7) functions as a thoracic vertebra; therefore neck movement is confined basically to five vertebrae.

Movement only in the anterior-posterior plane, that of flexion and

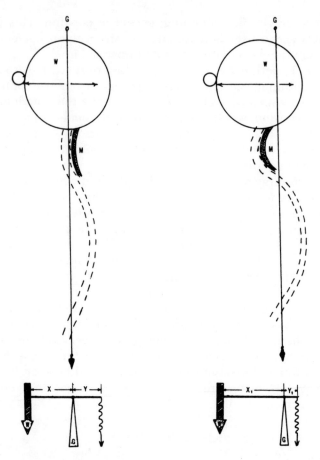

FIGURE 9. Gravity effect on a "forward head" posture with increased lordosis.

W = Weight of the head. Remains constant.
X = Distance of head weight (W) from center of gravity (G).
Y = Distance of spinal musculature from center of gravity (G).
M = Tension developed by musculature to sustain weight of head (W).

$$W \times X = M \times Y$$

In a simple lever system the weight supported by the fulcrum G is the sum of the weights acting at each end of the lever bar. Any change in the length of the lever bar must be compensated by a change in weight to maintain balance.

If W is 10 lbs. and distance X is 6″, the force exerted by M through lever arm Y of 4″ is 15 lbs.

If lever arm X increases to 8″, a forward shift of 2″, the weight of the head remains constant, the posterior lever arm Y decreases to 2″, and muscle tension must increase to 40 lbs. This increase not only is fatiguing but acts as a *compressive* force on the soft tissues including the disk.

12

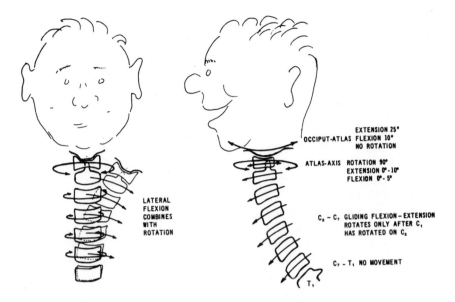

FIGURE 10. Composite movements of the cervical spine.

extension, occurs between the occiput and the atlas. This is the movement of "nodding" up and down in a sagittal plane. Flexion occurs in the range of 10 degrees and extension, 25 degrees.[2, 9, 10] The head can thus move a total of 35 degrees of flexion-extension without any neck participation (Fig. 11). All other movements between the skull and the atlas (C_1) are prevented by the direction of the opposing planes of the articular facets. In lateral flexion and rotation of the head and neck, the occiput (skull) and the atlas (C_1) move as one piece.

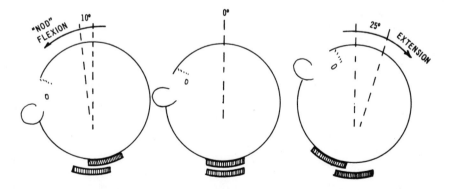

FIGURE 11. Occipital-atlas movement. Flexion-extension gliding of occiput on atlas in a "nodding" motion. No rotation or lateral flexion is possible.

The greatest movement of the entire cervical spine occurs between the atlas (C_1) and the axis (C_2). This articulation is termed the atlanto-epistrophic joint in the old terminology. Between these two vertebrae as much as 90 degrees of rotation is possible from the extreme right to extreme left (Fig. 12). Fifty percent of the total neck rotation occurs between C_1 and C_2 before any rotation is noted throughout the remainder of the cervical spine (between C_2 and C_7).

Some flexion and extension are possible between the atlas and the axis: as much as 10 degrees of extension and 5 degrees of flexion. Since the inferior facet of C_1 is flat and the opposing superior facet of C_2 is convex, flexion and extension at this level occur as a "rocker" action of C_1 on C_2.

Rotation of the second cervical vertebra (C_2) upon the third cervical vertebra (C_3) is mechanically limited by a bony locking mechanism in which the anterior tip of the upper articular process of the third cervical vertebra impinges upon the lateral process of the second cervical vertebra (Fig. 13). The lateral process of the vertebra is the lateral margin of the vertebral artery foramen. This locking mechanism prevents excessive rotation of the functional unit and thus protects the vertebral artery and the emerging nerve root in this specific intervertebral foraminal gutter.

Between C_2 and C_7, movements of flexion, extension, and lateral flexion rotation are possible. Flexion and extension occur as a "gliding" movement of the upper upon the lower vertebra. To permit this movement, the disk *distorts* horizontally and undergoes compression.

In the act of flexion, the anterior portion of the disk compresses and the posterior portion widens. The converse occurs during extension of

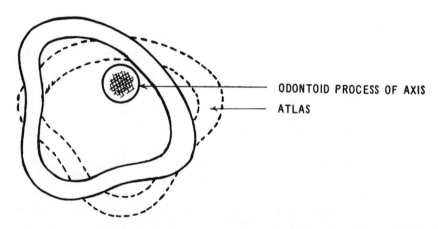

ODONTOID PROCESS OF AXIS
ATLAS

FIGURE 12.   Rotation of the atlas about the odontoid process of the axis (C_1 around C_2).

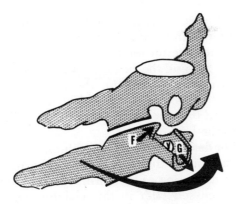

FIGURE 13.   Rotation of C_2 upon C_3 is limited by the mechanical locking of the articular structures. The anterior tip of the upper articular process of C_3 impinges upon the lateral margin of the foramen of the vertebral artery (V). G is the gutter through which emerges the nerve root of C_3.

the neck (Fig. 14). The longitudinal ligaments are sufficiently lax to permit this motion. As the posterior articulations also move in a similar gliding action, the capsules that enclose them must be elastic. In flexion the spinous processes separate as they correspondingly approach during extension. For adequate flexion and extension of the neck, flexibility of the connective tissues of the spine is an indispensable quality. Of clinical significance during flexion and extension is the opening of the intervertebral foramen with forward bending and narrowing of the foramen from extension (see Fig. 14).

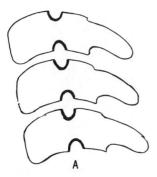
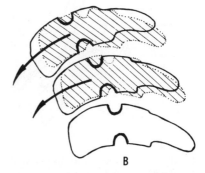

FIGURE 14.   "Gliding" movement in flexing spine from C_3 through C_7. A, Neutral position. B, Flexion with forward gliding, anterior disk compression, and widening posterior space.

15

In forward flexion the cervical canal lengthens, and in extension (dorsal flexion) it shortens. In flexion the posterior length of the canal elongates more than the anterior length, and the opposite occurs in extension (Fig. 15). In turning the head, rotation to left or right, the cervical canal also narrows, but in rotation the narrowing is caused by the dural action rather than bony narrowing. The dura, attached to the skull, twists on itself and *shutters* closed in its center as does a picture camera diaphragm in the lens opening.

There is no ascent or descent of the spinal column or the nerve roots within the spinal canal in flexing or extending the neck. There is merely a folding and unfolding of the cord, its dura, and the spinal nerves, as will be discussed later in this chapter under "Cervical Nerves."

Anterior-posterior movement occurs as a relatively pure motion. Lateral flexion and rotation never occur as isolated movements. Lateral flexion (side bending) always causes rotation, and rotation initiates lateral flexion. This axiom applies only to the cervical spine below the axis (C_2).

The foramina open on neck flexion and narrow on neck extension. They are influenced also by lateral bending and turning the head in that the foramina *close on the side to which the head laterally bends* and *toward which the head turns.* As lateral flexion and rotation occur simultaneously, the foramina close on the side *to* which the person turns his head. The converse happens in that the intervertebral

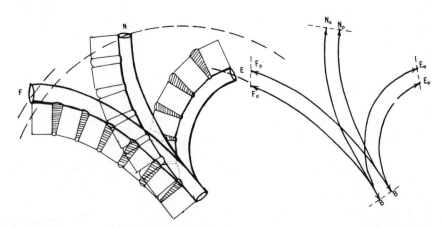

FIGURE 15. Alteration in spinal canal length. Length of neutral (N) spinal canal compared with that in flexion (F) and extension (E). In flexion the canal is longer and the anterior wall (F_a–B) is shorter than the posterior wall (F_p–B). In extension the total length of the canal is shorter, with the anterior wall (E_a–B) longer than the posterior wall (E_p–B). In neutral position both walls of the canal (N_a–B and N_p–B) are equal.

16

openings are increased on the side *from* which the head turns and away from which the head is tilted sideways (Fig. 16).

In a normal spine, the degree of narrowing of the foramen is not enough to compress any of the tissues contained within the foramina; so the flexion, extension, and rotation of the head leaves adequate room. In an abnormal spine in which the vertebrae come closer together or in which movement is excessive, the foramina understandably can become constricted.

The normal physiological *relationship of space to motion* in the cervical spine must be understood before the production of pain and

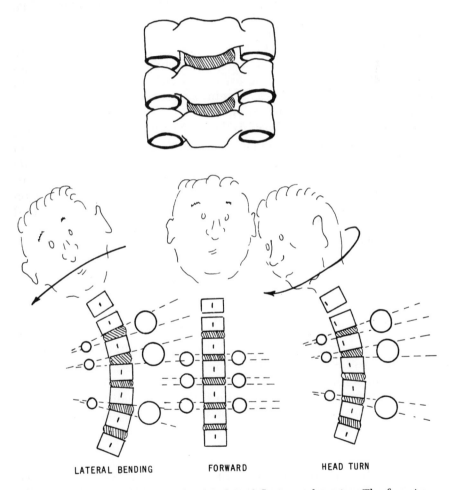

LATERAL BENDING   FORWARD   HEAD TURN

FIGURE 16.   Foraminal closure in head in lateral flexion and turning. The foramina close on the side toward which the head rotates or bends laterally, and they open on the opposite side.

17

dysfunction from impairment of movement and encroachment of space can be appreciated.

Clinical evaluation of the extent and site of flexion and extension of the neck introduces the factor of *sequence* in the act of bending the neck forward or backward. Flexion occurs to a large degree as a "nodding" motion of the occiput upon the atlas (C_1), and bending is a function of the remainder of the cervical spine. If the neck is fully flexed first then the chin is brought into flexion as a second phase, total neck flexion is less than if the chin is flexed first and followed by bending the rest of the neck. "Nodding" first (i.e., first flexing the chin then bending the neck) will result in a greater degree of total flexion[10] (Fig. 17).

Neck extension is slightly decreased in degree when the patient is standing. Flexion occurs at a lower level in the standing position than in the sitting position and at a slightly higher level when the chin is flexed first. These differences are more academically interesting than clinically significant, but the careful student and observer may note them in the clinical examination.

The cervical region C_4 to C_6 is the most active and most mobile. The greatest degree of flexion occurs in the midcervical region at the C_4 to C_5 and the C_5 to C_6 interspaces. Extension of the cervical spine is a more diffuse movement, but the site of maximum angulation is at the C_4 to C_5 interspace. There is great normal variation in the sites of maximum flexion and extension of the neck due to numerous factors that influence flexibility. Anatomical variations, soft tissue influences, and postural factors change the site of angulation. Maximum *movement*, whether flexion or extension, occurs in the region of C_4 to C_6; and as this is the region of maximum *static* curvature and thus maximum stress, it is evident that this portion has the most wear and tear.

LIGAMENTOUS SUPPORT

The ligaments of the neck are sufficiently resilient to control motion, thus aiding the support of the neck muscles; and they are lax enough to permit a great range of motion. Their resiliency is demonstrated by the protection they afford the spinal cord and the spinal nerves against the numerous stresses and strains accepted by the neck. The head is heavy and eccentrically balanced on a relatively narrow elastic support. In its top-heavy balance it is repeatedly subjected to movement, positional changes, and various degrees of trauma. The muscles and ligaments bear the brunt of these stresses, and the ligaments remain the sole support when the muscles are overpowered or fatigued.

The ligaments connecting the occiput to the atlas are extremely

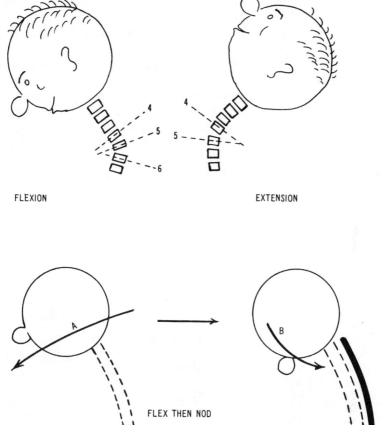

FLEXION   EXTENSION

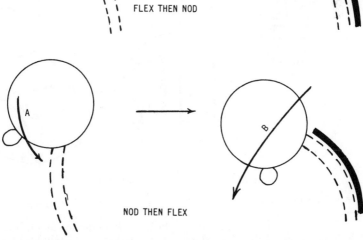

FLEX THEN NOD

NOD THEN FLEX

FIGURE 17. Influence of sequence upon neck flexion. Less total flexion occurs if neck first, then chin is flexed (nod). If chin is flexed first followed by neck flexion, there is greater total flexion.

dense and broad. These ligaments protect the entrance of the spinal cord through the foramen magnum into the skull and yet permit some 30 degrees of flexion and extension in a joint having no intervening disk and no posterior articulations.

The stability of the atlanto-axial (C_1 on C_2) joint is almost entirely dependent upon ligamentous structures. The atlas moves around the odontoid process and is firmly held to the process by the transverse ligament. This taut, resilient transverse ("cruciate" or "cruciform") ligament maintains the normal relationship of the atlas upon the axis, and a tear of this transverse ligament has the same result as a fracture of the odontoid process[11] (Fig. 18).

In the rest of the cervical spine from C_2 to C_7 the anterior and posterior longitudinal ligaments reinforce the disk annulus. The posterior longitudinal ligament is double layered and reinforces the cap-

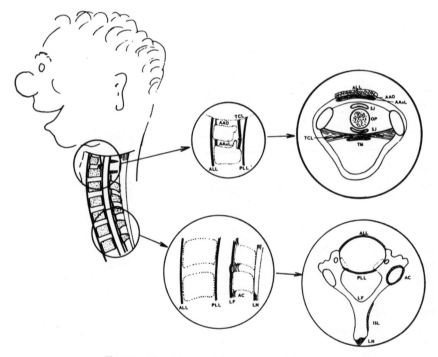

FIGURE 18. Ligamentous support of the neck.

OP	= Odontoid process	AAxL	= Atlanto-axial ligament
SJ	= Synovial joints	LF	= Ligamentum flavum
TCL	= Transverse cruciate ligament	PLL	= Posterior longitudinal ligament
TM	= Tectorial membrane (becomes posterior longitudinal ligament)	ALL	= Anterior longitudinal ligament
		AC	= Articular capsules
AAO	= Anterior atlanto-occipital ligament	ISL	= Interspinous ligament
		LN	= Ligamentum nuchae

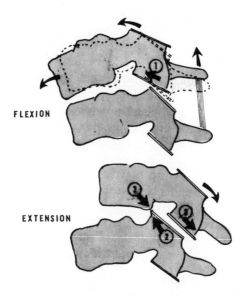

FIGURE 19. Translatory gliding on cervical flexion. The superior facet glides forward (1) and the essentially vertical facet elevates the posterior element until the interspinous ligament stops the movement. In extension, the superior facet glides posteriorly (3) until the inferior facet impinges upon the vertebra (2) and stops further extension.

sular ligaments. Combined, they limit the degree of transverse gliding motion between vertebrae as well as the extent of flexion and extension. Along the posterior wall of the spinal canal the ligamentum flavum combines with and reinforces the zygapophyseal joint capsules.

The posterior interspinous ligaments attached from the tips of adjacent posterior spinous processes limit the extent of flexion. As the cervical facets are essentially vertical, flexion is essentially movement in a vertical direction during forward flexion of the cervical spine. Flexion thus extends the posterior interspinous ligaments until they have reached their physiological limits, then they stop further movement (Fig. 19).

A broad, firm, fibrous posterior ligament attaches to the skull and connects the tips of the posterior spinous processes protectively against excessive flexion. This visible and easily palpable ligament is known as the ligamentum nuchae.

MUSCULATURE OF THE NECK

The neck muscles have been divided into two major functional groups: those that flex and extend the head (the so-called capital movers) and those that flex and extend the cervical spine[12] (Fig. 20).

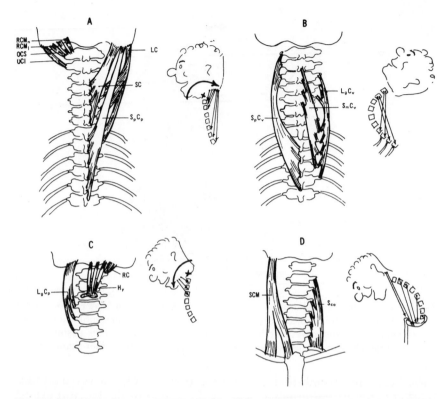

FIGURE 20. Musculature of the head and neck. *A* and *B*, The musculature of the extensor mechanism of the head and neck. *A*, The *capital extensors* attach to the skull and move the head upon the neck. *B*, The *cervical extensors* originate and attach upon the cervical spine and alter the curvature of the cervical spine. *C* and *D*, Flexion musculature. *C*, The *capital flexors* flex the head upon the neck. *D*, The *cervical flexors* attach exclusively upon cervical vertebrae and have no significant functional attachment to the skull.

RCM_n	= Rectus capitis minor	LC	= Longissimus capitis
RCM_j	= Rectus capitis major	SC	= Semispinalis capitis
OCS	= Obliquus capitis superior	S_pC_p	= Splenius capitis
OCI	= Obliquus capitis inferior	S_pC_v	= Splenius cervicis
L_gC_p	= Longus capitis	L_gC_v	= Longissimus cervicis
RC	= Rectus capitis anterior and lateral	S_mC_v	= Semispinalis cervicis
H_y	= Hyoideus and suprahyoid	SCM	= Sternocleidomastoid
	muscles	S_{ca}	= Scalene medius and anticus

The capital flexors are mainly the short recti and the longus capitis. The capital extensors are four short muscles extending from the base of the skull to the axis and atlas (*posterior rectus capitis minor* and *major* and the *obliquus capitis superior* and *inferior*) and longer muscles (*splenius capitis* and *splenius cervicis*) that are rotators sepa-

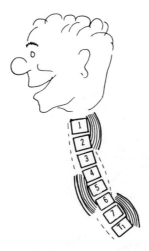

FIGURE 21. Sites of major muscle bulk in the cervical spine. The major bulk of extensor musculature in the head and neck is at the occipital-atlas-axis region and at the last cervical (C_6) thoracic articulations. These sites are the major points of stress. The major anterior (flexor) bulk is at the C_4–C_5 space, implying that the major flexion occurs here. This is also the site of maximum lordosis (curvature).

rately and extensors when working together bilaterally. Many other muscles, continuations of the total erector muscles of the vertebral column, affect the neck.

The main mass of neck muscle of the extensor group overlies the atlanto-axial area, which indicates this is the major site of stress. The bulk of flexor muscles centers at the fourth cervical vertebra (C_4), so this must be the site of maximum flexor stress (Fig. 21). In evaluating the mechanics of injury, stress upon and injury to the muscles is as important as stress upon and injury to the ligaments.

TISSUE SITES OF PAIN PRODUCTION

The neck contains many pain-sensitive tissues in a relatively small and compact area. Pain can result from irritation, injury, inflammation, or even infection of almost any of the contained tissues. Figure 22 depicts the tissues capable of causing pain and those considered pain insensitive.[13]

The cervical disk is stated to be a *non*sensitive tissue. The nucleus is an inert tissue in which no nerve tissue or nerve endings have been found.

Experimentally increased intradiskal pressure within a *normal intact* disk, such as a forceful injection of fluid into the disk, fails to cause

23

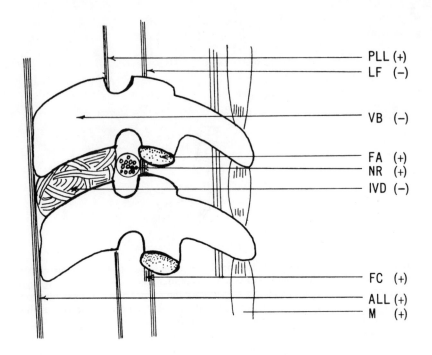

PLL (+)
LF (–)

VB (–)

FA (+)
NR (+)
IVD (–)

FC (+)
ALL (+)
M   (+)

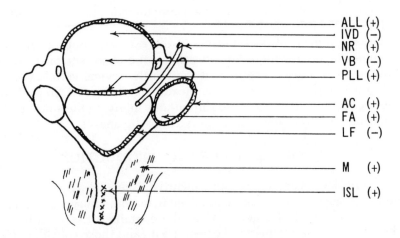

ALL (+)
IVD (–)
NR (+)
VB (–)
PLL (+)

AC (+)
FA (+)
LF (–)

M   (+)

ISL (+)

FIGURE 22. Tissue sites of pain production.

PLL = Posterior longitudinal ligament   IVD = Intervertebral disk
LF = Ligamentum flavum   FC = Facet capsule
VB = Vertebral body   ALL = Anterior longitudinal ligament
FA = Facet articulation   M   = Muscle
NR = Nerve root   ISL = Interspinous ligament

24

pain. Increasing pressure in a previously damaged or degenerated disk causes pain, but this pain can be abolished by locally anesthetizing the posterior longitudinal ligament. The posterior longitudinal ligament is innervated by fibers of the recurrent meningeal nerve of Luschka (Fig. 23). Pressure upon the ligament causes low back pain and possibly also causes neck pain.[14]

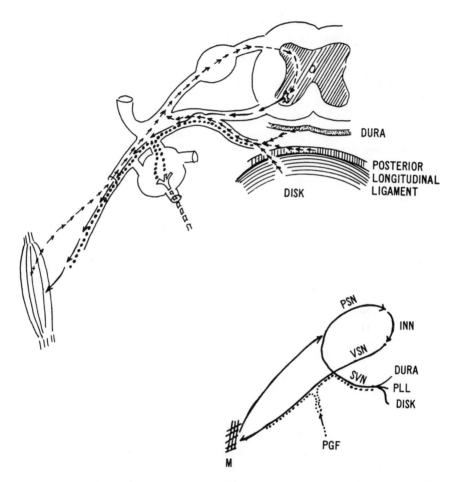

FIGURE 23. Postulated mechanism of "disk pain" (sciatica or brachialgia). The sinuvertebral nerve (SVN) originating or located in the annulus fibrosus (disk), in the longitudinal ligaments (PLL), or in the dura mater (dura) enters main nerve trunk and runs along the posterior spinal nerve (PSN). The arc to the anterior horn cell is via the internuncial nerve (INN), and the impulses leave along the ventral motor root (VSN) to the muscle (M), causing painful muscle spasm. This "myalgic" or sclerotomic pain returns via the sensory pathway back to the sensory root (PSN). As depicted in Figure 35, the sympathetic postganglionic fibers (PGF) accompany the sinuvertebral nerve (SVN) and the anterior primary ramus to the muscle.

The dural sleeve, not depicted in Figure 23, is shown later in Figures 26 and 32. The dura accompanies the nerve roots through the intervertebral foraminae to the outer margin of the foramen. The roots are enclosed essentially in a sleeve that contains spinal fluid and all the arterioles, venules, lymphatics, and fatty tissue.

The dura is also innervated by the recurrent nerve of von Luschka (also termed the sinuvertebral nerve).[14-17] Investigators of the sinuvertebral nerve cannot fully agree on the exact course and distribution of this nerve. There is no agreement as to whether or not it is the sensory nerve supply to the anterior longitudinal ligament.

The nerve root within the spinal canal and in its course through the intervertebral foramen is obviously a pain-sensitive tissue. Three sites are indicated in causing pain from nerve-root irritation: (1) the nerve fibers of the dural sheath of the nerve root; (2) involvement of the dorsal (sensory) root; and (3) the sensory fibers of the motor root. The mechanism of pain production remains unknown. Stretching the nerve and its dural sheath causes an impaired vascular circulation; so possibly ischemia causes the "nerve pain." "Pain is the cry of a nerve deprived of its blood supply," was aptly stated by Sir Henry Head.

The ligamentum flavum and the interspinous ligaments are nonsensitive to painful stimuli. The synovial lining of the posterior zygapophyseal joints is richly supplied with sensory and sympathetic vasomotor nerves. Apparently when these tissues are irritated, compressed, or otherwise inflamed, they can produce a distinctive and moderately severe pain. In spite of this assumption these joints in the cervical region *do not* seem to be a significant site and source of pain, since the degree of pain, limitation of motion, and disabling "stiffness" in their counterpart in the lumbar region is unrelated to the degree of change in the X-ray studies. Changes in the zygapophyseal joints, acute or chronic, undoubtedly cause pain in the neck region and participate in pain referred elsewhere by their influence on adjacent tissues. The capsular tissue around the joint is that most responsible for *"articular pain."* [18]

Pain can originate from muscle tissue in several ways. The concept that nerve root pressure causes a reflex muscle spasm which in turn causes the pain has been depicted in Figure 23. This concept places the pain and the tissue responsible in the neck musculature.

Pain can originate from ischemia of muscle. Sustained contractions can accumulate *work waste products* within the muscle while simultaneously constricting its intrinsic blood supply. These accumulated end-products of muscular contraction are irritating and play a part in the painful condition of *"cervical tension state."* [19]

Forceful muscle contraction as well as sustained contraction exerts traction at the myofascial junction to the periosteum, and the irritation

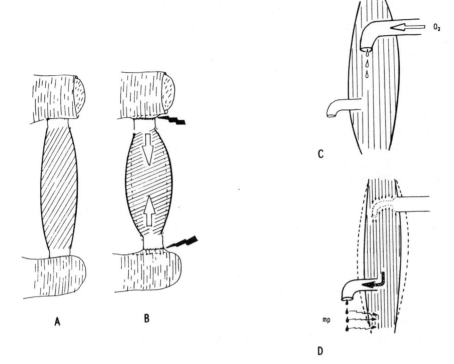

FIGURE 24. Pain production from myofascial-periosteal strain and muscle ischemia. A, Relaxed muscle with no traction upon its myofascial-periosteal attachment. B, The muscle contracted (shortened) with resultant traction stress upon the sensitive periosteum, causing pain and tenderness. C, Inflow of nutritive blood (O_2) into a relaxed muscle not forming waste products, mp. D, In the contracted muscle the source of oxygen is shut off, but the muscle is working and creating metabolic products irritating to muscle tissues. If D does not return to C and permit new blood to wash away mp and replenish the O_2 supply, the irritating mp cause pain.

of traction of the periosteum results in local pain and tenderness. In addition, movement passively stretching the muscle or movement actively contracting the muscle bellies results in pain. Small muscle fiber tears or tears of the fibrous elements within the muscles can have the same effects (Fig. 24).

THE CERVICAL NERVES

The cervical nerve is a mixed spinal nerve formed by the union of the anterior (ventral or motor) and the posterior (dorsal or sensory) roots that have emerged bilaterally from the cervical cord. The posterior and anterior spinal roots merge into a mixed nerve before enter-

27

ing the intervertebral foramen. Upon emergence from the interverte-bral foramen, the mixed nerve divides into two rami: the posterior ramus and the anterior ramus (Fig. 25).

The nerve fibers that coalesce into the nerve roots leave the cord at segmental sections at distances corresponding to the individual verte-brae. Each cervical nerve has a numerical designation correlating to corresponding cervical vertebra (Fig. 26). This correlation and desig-nation must be clarified, since it varies according to anatomical or clinical levels (Fig. 27).

No disk is between the occiput and the atlas (C_1) nor between the atlas (C_1) and the axis (C_2). The *first intervertebral disk* is between the axis (C_2) and the third cervical vertebra (C_3), at which foramen the C_3 nerve root emerges. With the physiological-anatomical classifica-tion, the third cervical nerve (C_3) is opposite the *first* intervertebral cervical disk. The conventional clinical nomenclature places the *first disk* between C_1 and C_2 vertebrae (where no intervertebral disk exists) and places the second cervical nerve root (C_2) at this point of emergence. This confusing situation is illustrated in Figure 27.

There are no intervertebral foramina between the occiput and the atlas and none between the atlas and the axis $(C_1$ and $C_2)$, so here, also, the correlation of specific nerve root in relationship to numbered foramen is not usable. The proper numbered nerve is related to its similar numbered vertebra rather than to the disk, disk space, or fora-men.

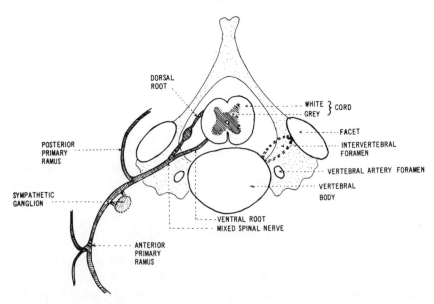

FIGURE 25. Component fibers of a cervical nerve.

After emerging from the cervical spinal cord, the nerve root fibers pass obliquely through the intervertebral foramen and down the foraminal groove (Fig. 28).

During forward (ventro) flexion, the cervical canal is lengthened so that the posterior wall elongates more than the anterior wall of the canal (see Fig. 15). The converse is true in extension (dorsal flexion), when the canal becomes shorter; in the fully extended position, the posterior wall of the canal shortens more than the anterior wall. In rotation of the head, the length of the canal is not influenced; but the cervical canal narrows, not from bony closure but from spiral motion of the dura.

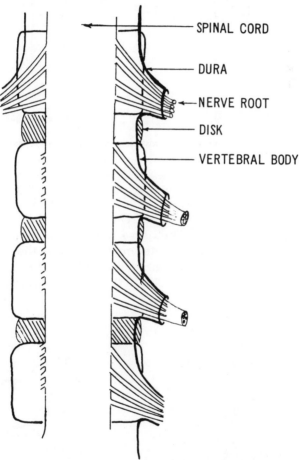

FIGURE 26. Formation and location of cervical nerve roots. The fila of the nerve roots emerge from the spinal cord at the level of the vertebral body, and the space between the group of fila that form the nerve roots is at the disk level. The relationship of nerve root to the disk is one of the reasons that disk herniation rarely impinges upon the nerve. The nerve root pierces the dura, and the dura accompanies the nerve as a sleeve.

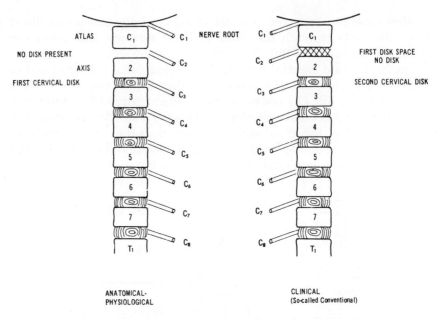

FIGURE 27. Nerve root location with regard to disk level.

The cord within the canal and its dura do not ascend or descend within the canal but on forward (ventro) flexion the cord and its dura elongate to their full *normal* length. On extension the dura folds as in accordion pleats (Fig. 29). The nerve roots are thought not to move within the foramina[20] during spine motion; rather they "move" because the cervical nerves become taut or relaxed during the elongation or folding of the dura (Fig. 30). In the neutral neck, and more so in

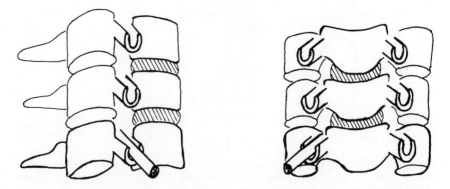

FIGURE 28.   Direction of foraminal grooves. Diagram depicting the downward-forward direction of the cervical nerve root.

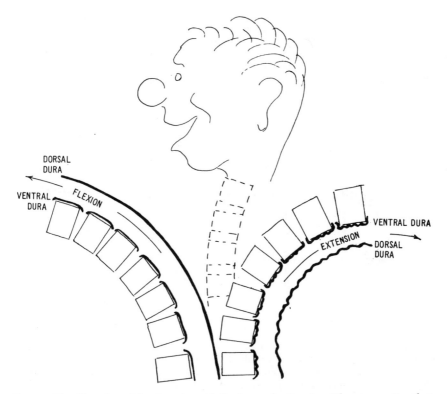

FIGURE 29. Reaction of the dura in neck flexion and extension. The assumption that the cord *ascends* in the canal during flexion and *descends* during extension (carrying the nerve roots with it, Fig. 30) is disproven. The dura becomes taut in physiological tension during flexion, thus "ironed out." In extension the dura folds, or pleats, and apparently "shortens." See text.

the flexed neck, the nerve roots are pulled taut within physiological tension and occupy an uppermost position in the intervertebral foramina, actually contacting the undersurface of the pedicle. As the neck extends (*dorsal flexion*), the cord dura relaxes and assumes a folded or corrugated appearance. The nerve roots also slacken and thus are more vertical to the cord; they descend in the foramen and lose contact with the undersurface of the pedicle above.

The nerve root is firmly anchored within the intervertebral foramen and does not glide within, in, or out of the foramen during this maneuver. Only if the foramen is narrowed or if there is acute inflammation or fibrosis within the foramen and the nerve root, is the nerve function impaired. As discussed, extension of the neck closes the foramina, so apparently the slackening of the nerve root tension in extension affords protection. Flexion, by increasing nerve root tension, brings the

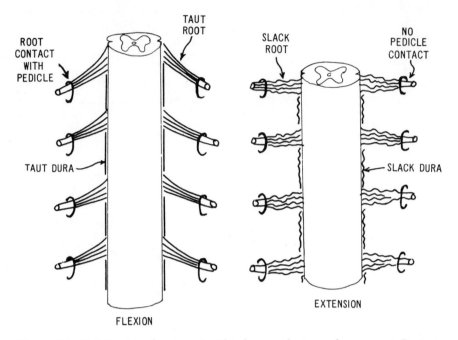

FIGURE 30. Relationship of nerve root within foramen during neck movement. During neck flexion (ventro flexion) the dura of the cord is pulled taut in physiological tension, and the nerve roots emerging from the lateral sulcus of the cord are also under tension. The nerve roots appear to ascend, but they merely become taut and occupy the upper portion of the foramen and contact the under-border of the pedicle above. In the extended position the dura pleats, as do the nerve roots; so the nerve is now slack, broader, but central in the foramen and away from the pedicle border.

nerve to the upper portion of the foramen; thus, in spite of a narrowed foramen, it is protected. Thus, pathology, to cause nerve deficit, must consist of *impairment of space* within the foramen, be it narrowing because of disk degeneration, anterior impingement due to spondylosis or disk herniation, posterior impingement because of facet inflammation or osteoarthritic changes, or compression of the nerve root because of inflammation or fibrosis within the nerve root sheaths.

Within the intervertebral foramen (Fig. 31) the nerve roots and their coatings are bounded superiorly and inferiorly (roof and floor) by the pedicles of the two opposing vertebrae. The pedicles belong to the vertebral arches included in the posterior portion of the functional unit (see Fig. 1).

The medial wall of the foramen is formed by the lateral aspect of the vertebral body and the joint of von Luschka. The zygapophyseal joints, formed by the superior and the inferior articular surfaces encased in their articular capsule, form the outer wall.

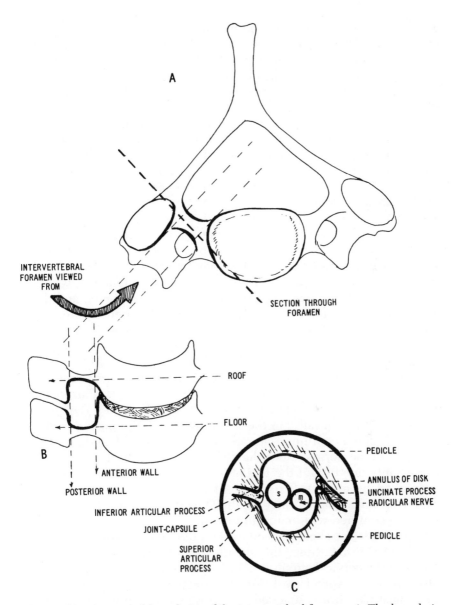

FIGURE 31. Anatomical boundaries of the intervertebral foramen. *A*, The boundaries of the foramen when viewed from the outside looking toward the spinal canal (large arrow) reveal the walls, roof, and floor as depicted in *B*. *C*, The mixed nerve (*s*, the sensory portion; *m*, the motor portion). The relationship of the sensory fibers to the posterior articulations and the relationship of the motor fibers to the joints of von Luschka and intervertebral disk are shown.

33

The mixed nerve proceeding along the foramen on its way out retains its isolated sensory and motor components. The motor or ventral root of the nerve is in intimate contact with the joint of von Luschka, and the sensory dorsal root lies close to the articular processes and their joint capsule (see Fig. 31). This relationship is clinically significant.[21]

The cervical nerve root normally occupies only one fifth to one fourth of the foramen. Its exact position and angulation through the foramen varies greatly. The angulation of the nerve is minimized and the nerve protected from traumatic sharp angulation by its coverings. Although these coverings protect the nerves, parodoxically they also contribute to pathology.

The nerve passing through the canal is enclosed within a funnel-shaped dural sac that tapers toward the intervertebral foramen. As they reach the entrance to the foramen, the nerve roots are separately enclosed in an arachnoid and a dural sleeve. Each sleeve is separated by the inter-radicular septum (Fig. 32). Lateral to the foramen, where the nerve enters the transverse process gutter, the arachnoid and the dura blend with the nerve sheath. The arachnoid layer ends here, and the nerve continues outward with merely the dural sheath. Because the arachnoid layer ends, the spinal fluid envelops the nerve only to and slightly past the interforaminal level[22] (Fig. 33).

Accompanying the *dura-arachnoid* coverings of the nerve root is a thin epidural membrane that contains small blood vessels. This membrane continues out through the foramen and becomes the periradicular sheath. Ventrally, in the foraminal canal, the posterior longitudinal ligament continues laterally as a fascial sheath and also becomes part of the periradicular sheath. Since the cervical nerve itself occupies only one fifth of the foramen, the remainder of the space is fully packed by many soft tissues. All these tissues are capable of inflammatory reaction and may swell. Thus the swelling and inflammation are confined within a rigid tunnel.

The periradicular sheath becomes the epineural sheath of the brachial plexus (Fig. 34). Since this sheath is firmly attached to the bony surfaces of the cervical spine, it helps prevent the nerves from being avulsed from the spinal cord during a traction injury.[22, 23] The epineural sheath is firmly attached to the transverse processes of the vertebrae and to the fascial prolongation of the posterior longitudinal ligament, and it has points of attachment to the scalene muscle group.

THE SYMPATHETIC NERVOUS SYSTEM

Two major components of the sympathetic nervous system are located in the neck. How these systems cause symptoms is neither fully

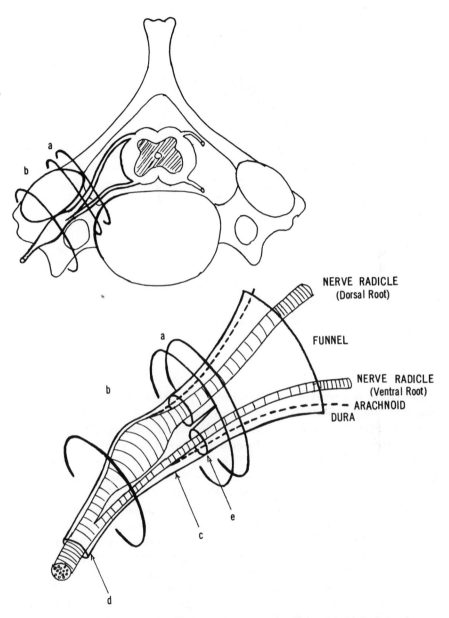

NERVE RADICLE
(Dorsal Root)

FUNNEL

NERVE RADICLE
(Ventral Root)

– – ARACHNOID

DURA

FIGURE 32.   Dura-arachnoid sleeve of nerve root in the intervertebral canal.

a = Intervertebral foramen
b = Gutter of the transverse process
c = At this point the arachnoid attaches to the dura and prevents spinal fluid from going further

d = Nerve from here on has only a dural coating
e = At apex of funnel, due to the inter-radicular septum, there are two ostia, one for the sensory and one for the motor roots

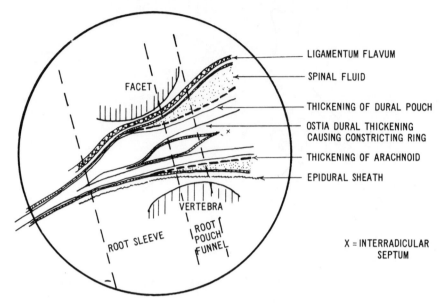

FIGURE 33. Cross section of contents of intervertebral canal: Root pouch funnel and root sleeve. See text.

understood nor universally accepted; but their presence is proven, and the symptoms attributed to them are accepted. These two components are the *sympathetic chain* and the *vertebral nerve*. The cervical spinal cord does not contain intermediolateral horn cells from which preganglionic fibers originate. The preganglionic fibers in the neck originate from intermediolateral horn cells in the thoracic spinal cord and ascend to the cervical ganglia (Fig. 35).

All cervical rami in the neck are *gray un*myelinated postganglionic nerves. They originate in the ganglia at the synapses with the ascending white preganglionic fibers from the thoracic area and go into three directions: (1) they accompany the anterior root along the posterior primary ramus and the anterior primary ramus of the peripheral nerve to the points of distribution of that nerve (see Fig. 35*A*); (2) they synapse into postganglionic fibers that pass to the eyes, the cranial nerves, the arteries of the head and neck, the subclavian arteries, and the cardiac plexus (see Fig. 35*B*); and (3) a branch enters back through the intervertebral foramen along the ventral root to communicate with the recurrent meningeal nerve that supplies the dura and interspinal canal ligamentous structures (see Fig. 35*C*). Other than the recurrent branch, all sympathetic nerve fibers are *extra*foraminal; they accompany peripheral nerves outside the intervertebral foramen.

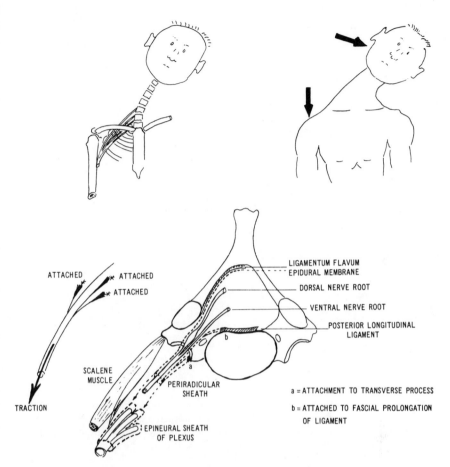

FIGURE 34. Periradicular sheath of nerve. The periradicular sheath is loose. It becomes adherent at the plexus level. The scalene muscles have points of attachment to the brachial plexus.

The second component of the sympathetic system in the cervical region is the *vertebral nerve* and the *vertebral plexus*. The vertebral nerve is thought to run along the vertebral artery, thus being contained in the arterial foramen of the cervical transverse processes. Irritation to this nerve is considered to occur from mechanical irritation to the vertebral artery anywhere along its course (Fig. 36).

Three types of symptoms are attributed to irritation of this vasomotor vertebral nerve (so-called Barré-Liéou syndrome[24]); namely, (1) vertiginous, (2) facial, (3) and pharyngeal. This syndrome can include headache, vertigo, tinnitus, nasal disturbance, facial pain, facial flushing, and pharyngeal paresthesias.

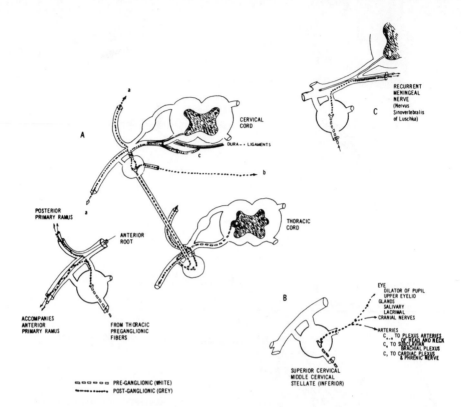

FIGURE 35. Sympathetic nervous system of the cervical region. The sympathetic fibers originate in the thoracic spine, as schematically depicted in the center figure. The grey (unmyelinated) fibers leave the ganglia and course in three directions: *A*, along the posterior primary rami and anterior primary rami; *B*, through the ganglia to the eye, cranial nerves, and arteries; and *C*, along the recurrent meningeal nerve. See text for detailed discussion.

Although sympathetic nerve fibers have never been found and confirmed anatomically along the cervical nerve roots within the intervertebral foraminal canal, surgical decompression of an entrapped nerve root has relieved symptoms attributed to the sympathetic nervous system as well as peripheral nerve symptoms. Relief of these symptoms by surgical decompression signifies the presence of either sympathetic nerve fibers, although as yet unproven, or a reflex mechanism, also as yet unexplained.

UPPER CERVICAL SEGMENTS

The upper two cervical functional units formed by the occiput and atlas and the atlas and axis are anatomically dissimilar from the functional units below (Fig. 37).

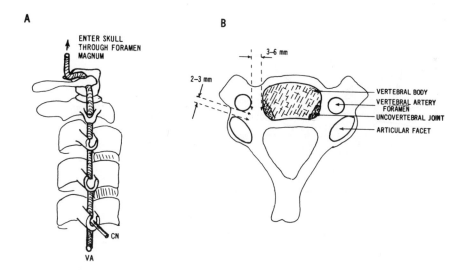

FIGURE 36. Vertebral artery pathway. *A*, The pathway of the vertebral artery as it ascends through the foramina. *B*, The relationship of the foramen to the vertebral body, the uncovertebral joint of von Luschka, and the zygapophyseal (facet) joint is evident. The space differences between body and foramen (3–6 mm) and facet foramen (2–3 mm) indicate that vascular impingement is most commonly due to encroachment by the superior articular process and rarely due to changes of the uncovertebral joints.

The first two cervical vertebrae, the atlas (C_1) and the axis (C_2), have *no* posterior articulations (facets or zygapophyseal joints) and there are *no* intervertebral foramina or funnels through which the cervical nerves emerge and travel.

The first two cervical nerves (C_1 and C_2) are primarily sensory. After leaving the spinal canal, they travel for the most part through soft connective tissue, mostly muscle. The sensory distribution of these nerves is the posterior and lateral portion of the scalp (see Fig. 37). Branches of C_3 join the first two branches in forming the greater and lesser occipital nerves. The sensory pattern extends forward to the frontal supraorbital area so that irritation of the nerves at the base of the skull can cause referred pain that mimics so-called "sinus trouble."

The nerves in this area are close to the vertebral artery at its point of angulation prior to entering the skull through the foramen magnum. These nerves are thus vulnerable to irritation and injury from the vertebral processes and from the myofascial attachment of the neck muscles to the base of the skull, muscles through which they traverse.

With the normal static and kinetic *neuro-musculo-skeletal* cervical spine established, deviations from normal that can cause pain and dysfunction can now be evaluated.

39

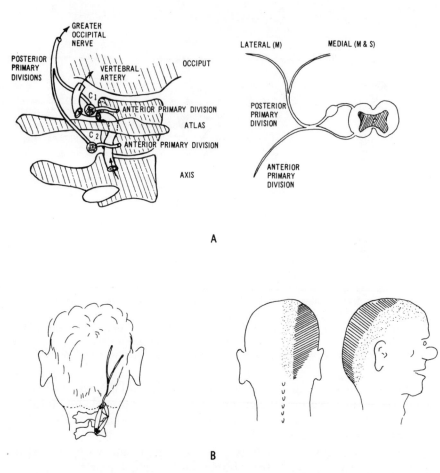

FIGURE 37. Upper cervical functional units (occipito-atlanto-axial). *A*, The course of the C_1 and C_2 nerves as they merge into the occipital nerve and their relationship to the vertebral artery in the atlas-axis region. *B*, Area (shaded) of hypasthesia, hyperesthesia, or anesthesia in the scalp area from pressure or irritation of these nerve roots.

REFERENCES

1. Armstrong, J. R.: Lumbar Disc Lesions. Edinburgh and London, Livingstone, 1952.
2. Fielding, J. W.: Cineroentgenography of the normal cervical spine. J. Bone Joint Surg. 39-A:1280–1, 1957.
3. Grant, J. C. B.: An Atlas of Anatomy, 5th ed. Baltimore, Williams & Wilkins, 1962.
4. Orofino, C., Sherman, M. S., and Schechter, D.: Luschka's joint—A degenerative phenomenon. J. Bone Joint Surg. 42-A:853–8, 1960.
5. Stedman's Medical Dictionary. Baltimore, Williams & Wilkins, 1976.
6. Hadley, L. A.: The Spine: Anatomico-Radiographic Studies, Development and the Cervical Region. Springfield, Ill., Charles C Thomas, 1956.

7. Jackson, R.: The Cervical Syndrome, 2d ed. Springfield, Ill., Charles C Thomas, 1958.
8. Schneider, R. C. and Crosby, E. C.: Vascular insufficiency of brain stem and spinal cord in spinal trauma. Neurology 9:643–56, 1956.
9. Werne, S.: The possibilities of movement in the cranio-vertebral joints. Acta Orthop. Scand. XXVIII:165–73, 1959.
10. Jones, M. D.: Cineradiographic studies of the normal cervical spine. Cal. Med. 93:293–6, 1960.
11. Netter, F. H.: The Ciba Collection of Medical Illustrations, vol. I: The Nervous System. Summit, N. J., Ciba Pharmaceutical Products, 1957.
12. Perry, J. and Nickel, V. L.: Total cervical-spine fusion for neck paralysis. J. Bone Joint Surg. 41-A:37–60, 1959.
13. Inman, V. T. and Saunders, J. B. de C. M.: Referred pain from skeletal structures. J. Nerv. Ment. Dis. 99:660–7, 1944.
14. Herlihy, W. F.: Sinu-vertebral nerve. New Zealand Med. J. 48:214–216, 1949.
15. Jung, A. and Brunschwig, A.: Recherches histologique sur l'innervation des articulations des corps vertebraux. Prese Med. 40:316–317, 1932.
16. Roofe, R. P.: Innervation of annulus fibrosus and posterior longitudinal ligament, fourth and fifth lumbar level. Arch. Neurol. Psychiat. 44:100–103, 1940.
17. Weiberg, G.: Back pain in relation to the nerve supply of the intervertebral disk. The Orthopedic Clinic, Lind, Sweden. Acta Orthop. Scand. 19:213, 1941.
18. Cyriax, J. H.: Text-book of Orthopaedic Medicine, vol. I.: Diagnosis of Soft Tissue Lesions. London, Paul B. Hoeber, 1954.
19. Dorpat, T. L. and Holmes, T. H.: Mechanisms of skeletal muscle pain and fatigue. A. M. A. Arch. Neurol. Psychiat. 74:528–40, 1955.
20. Breig, A.: Biomechanics of the Central Nervous System. Chicago, Year Book Publishers, 1960.
21. Teng, P.: Spondylosis of the cervical spine with compression of the spinal cord and nerve roots. J. Bone Joint Surg. 42-A:392–407, 1960.
22. Frykholm, R.: Cervical nerve root compression resulting from disc degeneration and root-sleeve fibrosis: A clinical investigation. Acta Chir. Scand. Supp. 160, 1951.
23. Barcroft, H. and Dornhurst, A. C.: The blood flow through the human calf during rhythmic exercise. J. Physiol. 109:402–11, 1949.
24. Barré, M.: Sur un syndrome sympathetique cervicale posterieur et sa cause frequent: L'Arthrite cervicale. Rev. Neurol. 33:1246–8, 1926.

BIBLIOGRAPHY

Cloward, R. B.: Lesions of the intervertebral disk and their treatment by interbody fusion method. Clin. Orthop. 27:51–77, 1963.
——————: Anterior herniation of a ruptured lumbar invertebral disk: Comments on the diagnostic value of diskogram. A. M. A. Arch. Surg. 64:457–63, 1952.
Steindler, A.: An analysis and differentiation of low-back pain in relation to the disk factor. J. Bone Joint Surg. 29:455–60, 1947.

CHAPTER 2

Neck Pain Originating in the Soft Tissues

To know the normal and to recognize deviation from normal; to be able to reproduce the pain by reproducing the abnormal position or movement; to understand the mechanism by which the pain is caused—this is the formula for clinically evaluating the patient complaining of pain and dysfunction of the neck, shoulder, and upper extremity.

Pain in and from the neck region is variously described and originates from many tissue sites. Pain is produced by many different mechanisms. It can be felt directly in the neck, or it can originate in the neck and be felt elsewhere. The numerous tissues in the neck capable of causing pain have already been shown in Figure 22.

Frequently pain is not felt at its origin. Pain originating in bone or skin is felt at its source, but pain originating in other deep somatic structures is more vague and diffuse in its distribution and may be referred to a distal site.

Neck and head pain can originate in the muscles of the neck. So-called *cervical tension state* and *tension headaches* occur in the neck and the head as a direct result of sustained muscular contraction. There are several mechanisms by which pain is produced by muscular tension.

Pain may occur at the periosteal site of muscular attachment. Most of the neck muscles do not terminate in tendons but attach to the bone by myofascial tissue that blends into the periosteum. Traction exerted upon the periosteum can cause pain and tissue tenderness. Sustained muscle contraction, such as occurs in emotional tension or in maintaining an awkward posture for prolonged periods, will produce sustained traction at the site of insertion (see Fig. 24). An acute muscle contraction or ligamentous stretch, such as in an accident or quick movement of the head, can cause an acute traction with resultant irritation at the periosteal site of attachment. Either acute or sustained

42

traction upon these pain-sensitive tissues can cause local pain or tenderness. A common site of this local tenderness is at the base of the skull, in the occiput, where the neck extensor muscles attach and cause the common "tension headache at the base of the skull." The muscles attach to the occiput at the site of emergence and passage of the superior occipital nerve, which when irritated will transmit and refer pain across the top and side of the scalp to the frontal area (see Fig. 37).

Pain and tenderness can occur within the belly of the muscle as a result of contraction, either acute or sustained. Muscle contraction creates intramuscular pressure.[1] Intramuscular pressures are significantly greater in *isometric* contraction (a muscle contracted but prevented from shortening) than in *isotonic* contraction (a muscle permitted to shorten or contract when stimulated). Collapse of small blood vessels and tears of muscle fibers have been demonstrated to result from strong isometric contractions.

Acute, simultaneous contraction of all the neck muscles resulting from trauma can cause excessive intramuscular pressure with or without muscle tear. The end result of increased internal pressure is inflammation and leads to "myositis," a painful condition.[2] This is part of the muscular component of acute cervical strain from the commonly called "whiplash" injury.

Sustained muscular contraction in a static neck results in *tension myositis*. All the neck muscles contract simultaneously, in *isometric* contraction. Whatever the cause of the muscular tension, be it emotional tension from fear or anxiety or faulty neck position from posture or occupation, the cause of pain is *ischemia*.[3, 4] The adjective *tense* denotes "being drawn tightly or taut." To become taut, a muscle must contract. During contraction, the internal pressure of the muscle belly increases, constricting the blood vessels and stopping internal circulation. The contracted muscle is performing work, thus creating metabolites, which requires oxygen.

Severe muscular exercise is known to cause pain that may persist for several hours after the cessation of the exercise.[5] A "fatigue curve" has been experimentally demonstrated by sensitive electromyography (EMG) indicating a decrease in the amplitude of the maximum voluntary contraction and an inability of the muscle fibers to relax.

This latter phenomenon is attributed to irritability of the spindle cells. Once the muscle fibers are fully contracted (by muscular effort) they do not automatically (reflexly) relax and thus by remaining contracted, cause persistence of intramuscular pressure. This sustained pressure causes increased ischemia *and* further production of metabolites which in turn cause further irritation and thus further muscle contraction. A vicious cycle results.

43

It is well accepted in sports medicine that sustained stretching of the affected muscle to its full length and maintaining this stretched position for a period of at least two minutes results in diminution or cessation of pain.[6] This is attributed to the reflex inhibition of muscular contraction originating in the tendon Golgi apparatus. The amplitude of the EMG diminishes in large muscles when they are stretched.[7] The tendon receptor organs (Golgi) can inhibit the entire muscle contraction when intiated or stimulated.

"Cramps," a form of muscle contraction, differ from voluntary muscular activity yet have some similarity. There are some who claim that "cramps" are essentially a discharge of a motor unit, but in a cramp there are synchronous discharges of other adjacent motor units therefore *it is more probable* that cramps are caused by spinal (rather than peripheral) excitability albeit merely an exaggeration of normal muscular activity.[8]

Discharge or irritation of the spinal reflex can be due to an afferent stimulus such as a painful sensory stimulus or a normal sensory stimulus affecting an already irritable central nervous reflex arc.

Relief of cramps by lengthening the muscle may do so by the reflex mechanism of the Golgi apparatus (Fig. 38). By stretching the tendon, the Golgi system causes central reaction which "unloads" the spindle cells and allows the muscle fibers to relax.

It is paradoxical that the muscle shuts off its own blood supply when it needs oxygen and blood flow to wash out the metabolites it creates. Physiologically, every period of work (contraction) must be followed by a period of relaxation during which blood again flows through the released capillary beds bringing in new oxygen and removing the accumulated waste products.[9] Alternating contraction and relaxation permits painless, nonfatiguing muscular activity. Sustained muscle contraction upsets this normal cycle. Work continues with impaired circulation, thus with inadequate oxygenation and faulty removal of waste products. *Ischemic* muscle pain results.

Ischemic muscle pain results not only from lack of oxygen. Irritating metabolites such as "Factor P,"[10] potassium shift,[11] or lactic acid accumulation[12] within the muscle are considered to produce pain. The combination of tissue ischemia and retained metabolites initiates a tissue *inflammation* that leads ultimately to fibrous reaction within the muscles and their contiguous tissues. Thus a cycle toward pain and disability results (Fig. 39).

Pain can originate in the joints of the neck, but *arthritic* pain in the neck is far less significant and prevalent than the frequent clinical diagnosis of "pain due to cervical arthritis" would imply. The painful manifestation of *osteoarthritis*[13] probably is due to capsular thickening with its resultant limited joint movement. Stretching these

44

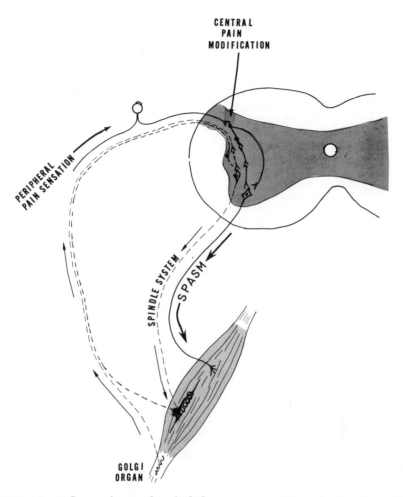

FIGURE 38. Reflex mechanism for relief of cramps: concept. Lengthening the tendon stimulates the Golgi apparatus that reflexly "unloads" the spindle system causing the extrafusal muscle fibers to relax.

thickened and contractured periarticular tissues on attempted neck movements causes the pain felt in the neck. That these contracted tissues can cause pain when they are stretched is ascertained by the decrease in pain when the capsular contractures have been elongated by stretching exercises. The decrease in painful movement is accompanied by an increase in joint range of motion with no obvious change in the degeneration in the neck.

Marked erosion of the cartilage of the synovial joints of the neck with roughening of the opposing articular surfaces may cause a sensation and sound of "grating," but grating is unrelated to pain.

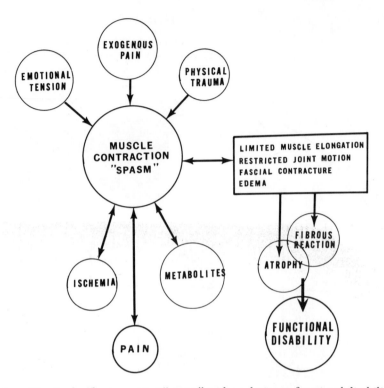

FIGURE 39. Cycle of pain causing "spasm" with evolution to functional disability.

There is little or no correlation between the degree of pain felt in the neck and the degree of arthritic changes found on X-rays. Symptomatic osteoarthritis is a clinical diagnosis in which range of motion is limited and pain results from exceeding the limits of motion. The clinical findings are usually associated with some significant changes in the X-ray but not always to a degree equivalent to the symptoms.

A neck condition that may be associated with pain and with some degree of disability is torticollis (*L. tortus,* twisted; *collum,* neck), a scoliosis of the cervical spine that may be caused by many conditions. In children, torticollis may result from trauma, or it may be secondary to infection of the throat, pharynx, or cervical adenitis. In its more severe form the adenitis may cause a softening of the odontoid ligaments and place the spinal cord in jeopardy from any acute movement.[14] Torticollis in the adult may result from a viral infection, a muscular strain, a psychogenic etiology, or a traumatic subluxation of a unilateral apophyseal joint. In a ligamentous strain with some degree of subluxation, movement is further limited by the muscles acting protectively, but motion should return with time and simple therapeutic measures.

Psychogenic torticollis is a habit spasm, a psychoneurotic *tic* that expresses a turning away from an emotional conflict.[15] This diagnosis can tax the diagnostic acumen and exhaust the therapeutic skills of the most astute physician. The emotional etiology is suggested by the bizarre findings in both the history and the physical examination of a patient with known or suspected emotional problems. The subjective claims are out of proportion to the objective findings, and relief for any duration by physical and medical measures fails. The physician who recognizes psychoneurotic symptoms should direct the patient to psychiatric treatment, thus preventing unnecessary, prolonged treatment or surgery that would merely intensify the torticollis and further "fix" the psychological abnormality.

Torticollis, or "wry neck," can result from unilateral facet subluxation or impingement. In a fully flexed, fully extended, or fully rotated position, the posterior neck joints are normally at the *verge of subluxation*. The ligamentous and capsular tissues prevent their exceeding the limits of normal movement. Forward or backward subluxation will be considered in subsequent chapters, but torticollis can occur from *rotatory subluxation.*

Abrupt or excessive turning of the head may cause one or more pairs of facets to move past their normal range of motion. To pass this point requires excess stretching of capsular tissue and elongation of ligaments. At this point, the articular surfaces lose their normal relationship and the two joints on the side to which the head is tilted and towards which it is turned "jam" together and the joints on the opposite side separate (Fig. 40). Pain results from (1) capsular stretch and

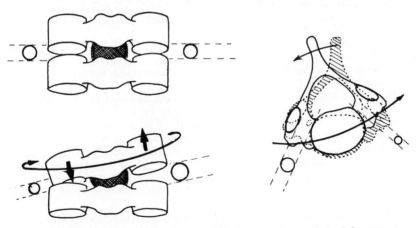

FIGURE 40. Unilateral subluxation from excessive rotation (unilateral facet impingement or dislocation).

tear, (2) synovial impingement with swelling of the synovial membrane and capsular structure, and (3) foraminal encroachment upon the nerve root and other tissues contained therein by swelling facets and unilateral narrowing of the foramen.

Exceeding the impingement stage results in subluxation which not only causes disruption of the articular positions but alters the spinal canal and the vertebral artery foraminal alignment. Thus, damage to the spinal cord, to the peripheral nerves, and to the vertebral arteries may occur. Further consideration will be given to *subluxation* in a subsequent chapter.

Neck pain originating in the soft tissues of the neck and felt in the neck cannot exclude *disk pain*. The intervertebral disk plays a vital part in the normal mechanism of the neck and is involved to some degree in all neck pain, whether the pain is felt locally, distally, or both. It merits more exhaustive consideration.

REFERENCES

1. Hill, A. V.: The pressure developed in muscle during contraction. J. Physiol. 107:518–26, 1948.
2. Neufeld, I.: Mechanical factors in the pathogenesis, prophylaxis, and management of fibrositis (fibropathic syndromes). Arch. Phys. Med. Rehab. 36:759–65, 1955.
3. Barcroft, H. and Millen, J. L. E.: The blood flow through muscle during sustained contraction. J. Physiol. 97:17–31, 1939.
4. Anrep, G. V. and Von Saalfeld, E.: Blood flow through the skeletal muscle in relation to its contraction. J. Physiol. 85:375–99, 1935.
5. deVries, H. A.: Quantitative electromyographic investigation of the spasm theory of muscle pain. Am. J. Phys. Med. 45:119–34, 1966.
6. deVries, H. A.: Prevention of muscular distress after exercise. Res. Quart. 32:177–85, 1961.
7. Morris, F. H., Gasteiger, E. L., and Chatfield, P. O.: An electromyographic study of induced and spontaneous muscle cramps. Electroencephalogr. Clin. Neurophysiol. 9:139–77, 1957.
8. Thomas, A. and Ajieriaguerra, J.: Les etats de grande hypertonie. Etude Semiologigue du Tonus Musculaire Flammarion, Paris, 1949.
9. Barcroft, H. and Dornhurst, A. C.: The blood flow through the human calf during rhythmic exercise. J. Physiol. 109:402–11, 1949.
10. Perlow, S., Markle, P., and Katz, L. N.: Factors involved in the production of skeletal muscle pain. Arch. Int. Med. 53:814–24, 1934.
11. Baetjer, A. M.: The diffusion of potassium from resting skeletal muscles following reduction in blood supply. Am. J. Physiol. 112:139–46, 1935.
12. Katz, L. N., Lindner, E., and Landt, H.: On the nature of the substance(s) producing pain in the contracting skeletal muscle: Its bearing on the problems of angina pectoris and intermittent claudication. J. Clin. Invest. 14:807–21, 1935.
13. Tarsy, J. M.: Pain Syndromes and Their Treatment. Springfield, Ill., Charles C Thomas, 1952, p. 35.
14. Grisel, P.: Enucléation de l'atlas et torticolis nasopharynien. Presse Med., 38 (Jan. 1930), 50–53. Quoted and reviewed by A. W. Davis: Post-infectious, non-traumatic atlanto-axial subluxation or dislocation (Grisel's syndrome). Unpublished paper

presented at Pediatric Meeting, Los Angeles County General Hospital, April 17, 1956.

15. Bauer, J.: Differential Diagnosis of Internal Diseases: Clinical Analysis and Synthesis of Symptoms and Signs on Pathophysiologic Basis. New York, Grune and Stratton, 1955, p. 327.

CHAPTER 3

Diagnosis of Neck Pain

Knowing normal and recognizing deviation from normal clarifies the mechanism of pain production and indicates correct treatment. Numerous chapters will discuss the normal cervical spine and pathological changes in the component parts of the neck. The method of history taking, its significant revelations, and the confirmation by examination should be apparent. Only salient points that need emphasis will be elaborated here.

When there has been no obvious trauma, the cause of neck pain may have been an unaccustomed exertion, an awkward position, or a prolonged posture not fully understood by the patient until revealed by careful questioning. Examples of stressful positions or activities include ceiling painting, storing objects in overhead cupboards, lying prone with the head elevated in reading or watching television, or doing a usual job while under unusual emotional pressures.

Emotional tension as an etiological factor of neck pain must be fully understood. The musculoskeletal dynamics of pain, rather than merely the psychodynamics, enter into the picture. The emotional state of man as depicted in his posture has a definite influence on the neck, both in curvature and in relationship to center of gravity. The round-shouldered posture of the depressed individual must be compensated by an increase in cervical lordosis. The forward position of the head causes an increase in muscle tone to maintain the eccentrically placed head. The hostile, aggressive person often centers his tension in the neck muscles.

Prolonged or intensive tension causes (1) painful "tension myositis" on an ischemic basis, (2) increase in myostatic contracture as an adaptive shortening of the fibrous elements of the muscle, which, when stretched, is painful, (3) myofascial stretch irritation of the periosteum at the point of insertion, (4) thickening of the facet capsules from a failure to undergo periodic elongation, and (5) persistent compression of the disk that ultimately must be detrimental to its nutrition. Merely recognizing the presence of "tension" and diagnosing "psychogenic factors" does not deny the advisability of treating the secondary manifestations in the soft tissues.

PHYSICAL EXAMINATION

Physical examination has already begun while watching the posture and attitude of the patient during history taking. Posture observed while the patient is unaware compared to that noted while being examined may well reveal the true posture contrasted to what the patient wishes to portray or considers as the proper posture.

The kinetic neck examination is exacting and revealing, as well as difficult to record on a history-physical chart. Range of motion, active and passive, must be judged and reproduction of pain noted. Active flexion done with "chin-in" first then total flexion followed by "chin-in" is observed for the extent of bending as revealed in the *degree of reversal of cervical lordosis*. Extension with and without rotation, the cause of pain in most instances, is also tested. After the physician observes the active range of motion, he tests the same range passively. Limitation of these motions, as well as the direction of limited movement, reflect the restrictions imposed by the soft tissues: the ligaments, capsules, and muscles that surround the disks and the posterior joints.

Lateral flexion and rotation occur simultaneously in the lower cervical spine. Ninety degrees of rotation are possible between C_1 and C_2 before any rotation occurs below these segments, so obviously active and passive restriction of rotation must be evaluated with this in mind. Neither lateral flexion nor rotation occur between the skull and the atlas, and very little lateral flexion occurs at the atlanto-axis joint; evidently testing lateral flexion tests the flexibility of the lower cervical spine. Lateral flexion is tested by bringing the ear *to* the shoulder; rotation, by bringing the chin *to* the shoulder. It is extremely easy for the patient with tight tissues to elevate unwittingly the shoulder to the ear or chin and give an erroneous impression of normal range of motion; thus painful neck movements are avoided by substituting shoulder movements. During the examination, preventing this shoulder motion may reveal the limited and the painful neck motion.

Motor weakness or fatiguability of musculature can be determined by resisting the basic motions of flexion, short and long; extension, short and long; lateral flexion; and rotation. Gross inequalities will be evident. Atrophy or palpably thinner muscles confirm the site of weakness.

Neurological examination requires testing the presence and bilateral symmetry of the deep tendon reflexes. Pin scratch evaluation of the dermatome patterns helps determine a specific site of lesion. A careful motor test of the upper extremities is an invaluable part of the neurological examination. The specific localizing neurological signs are depicted later in the text in Figures 49, 50, and 51.

The above symptoms are predominantly lower motor neuron signs; and since cervical spine pathology may cause cord damage, the examination must include testing for the Babinski and Hoffman signs, vibration and position sense, and coordination test of cerebellar function. Testing the cranial nerves completes the clinical neurological examination and indicates the need for more thorough studies. The exact level of nerve root involvement cannot be specifically localized by motor or sensory examination alone since overlapping of innervation clouds the issue.

X-RAY EXAMINATION

Interpretation of the X-rays must be considered as adjunctive to a clinical evaluation and per se is rarely the sole basis for diagnosis.

Congenital abnormalities are only rarely responsible for symptoms; but when they are, they may cause serious and even fatal neurological damage. The site and extent of the defect must be anatomically determined and correlated with any existing neurological signs and symptoms. The possibility of a defect causing symptoms after an injury confuses the medical-legal situation, much to the consternation of all involved.

Fractures and dislocations of the cervical spine demand early and accurate diagnosis so that, if they are recognized, treatment can be instituted *to produce a stable, painless neck* and *prevent or diminish pressure on the spinal cord* or nerves. Here proper treatment is dictated by the X-ray.

The initial X-ray of an injured neck must limit the number of views so as to minimize neck manipulation on the X-ray table. An initial lateral view will reveal an unstable dislocation of the cervical spine. If a vertebral body has dislocated *less* than half the width[1] of the vertebra below (A-P width), only one facet has dislocated, and the dislocation is reasonably stable (i.e., usually does not displace further). Which side or which facet is dislocated can then be determined by oblique views.

Forward dislocation of *more than half* the A-P width of the vertebral body below indicates that both facets are dislocated, indicating tearing of the longitudinal, interspinous, and facet ligaments as well as of the disk annulus. These are unstable dislocations and must be treated so as not to compound the injury.

Stable fractures are those in which the posterior ligamentous structures remain intact. *Instability* results from tears of the posterior ligaments. In stable fractures, reduction and immobilization are not necessary for good results, whereas in the unstable ones, reduction, immobilization, and, frequently, fusion are necessary. Failure to recognize fractures or dislocations and to determine stability or instability can permit serious damage to the enclosed nervous tissues, the cord, and the spinal nerve roots, by direct pressure or vascular occlusion.

Extension dislocations in the cervical spine are frequent and are often missed on X-rays, since they tend to reduce spontaneously. Because the posterior ligaments remain intact, the dislocation is *stable*. Tear of the anterior longitudinal ligament must occur to permit significant posterior (extension) dislocation; this may be evidenced merely by a small avulsion fracture of the anterior edge of the vertebral body. Anterior separation resulting from flexion injury usually produces separation of the spinous processes seen on the lateral view.

True X-ray evaluation of the cervical spine can be done only by taking *all* views. These views include (1) anterior-posterior views, (2) open-mouth view for visualization of the atlas-axis region, (3) lateral views, and (4) both oblique views. Lateral views in full flexion and in full extension may sometimes reveal a subluxation not otherwise evident, but full agreement regarding the interpretation of these views is not yet standardized. Cinematoradiology, to view the sequence of flexion and extension, has research value and may ultimately be used clinically.

Myelography (pantopaque dye studies) views the contour of the dural canal, to a degree the patency of the nerve sleeves, the posterior extension of the disk and bony protrusions into the spinal canal, and the subdural space around the cord within the bony canal. The test has a surprisingly limited value since it is altered by neck positions, does not flow far enough to show intraforaminal prominences, and many protrusions seen on myelography are asymptomatic.[2] Controlled comparative studies revealed that the *same* percentage of patients *without symptoms* had medium or large protrusion as did patients *with symptoms*. The level of the dye defect is not always at the clinical level. Again, it must be emphasized that any laboratory test must be carefully judged in the light of the history and of the physical examination.

Diskography is a diagnostic roentgenographic test in which contrasting dye material is injected *into the disk*[3] to picture the integrity of the annulus and the nucleus and to demonstrate the presence of defects or damage to either. A normal diskogram indicates an intact annulus with a well contained nucleus. Finding a normal disk is of

53

value especially if a subsequent diskogram is found abnormal. The intervening history may be incriminated in the cause of the damage.

The present controversy is in the interpretation and significance of abnormal diskograms and the relevance of these abnormal findings to the symptoms and findings elicited clinically. What does an abnormal diskogram tell, and how does it correlate with the clinical findings? The answer to these questions at present is disappointing.[4]

Very few normal diskograms are found in people over 25 years old who may or may not have symptoms. Abnormal disks are found in increasing frequency and severity with increasing age, so that by age 60 *no* cervical disks are found to be normal. Evidently the progressive disk degeneration found with aging[5, 6] reveals an abnormal diskogram but is obviously unrelated to clinical symptoms, since many older people are free of symptoms referable to cervical disk disease.

Injection of material into a disk may reproduce the patient's symptoms, thus localizing the offending disk. The material so injected can be saline and need not produce an abnormal X-ray picture. Therefore a *diskometric* test affords the information, not the *diskogram*. A normal disk permits only a small amount of fluid to be injected before resistance is met. A degenerated disk will allow much more fluid to enter and ultimately will cause symptoms. If the symptoms reproduce the clinical picture, the specific disk is localized. If the disk allows the entrance of more fluid with no reproduction of symptoms, all that is learned is that the disk is degenerated or damaged. The value of this test is obviously questionable.

To discourage further the routine use of this test, it can be added that (1) the test is technically difficult, (2) there is discomfort to the patient, (3) there is difficulty clinically determining *which* disk to inject, and (4) it has not been conclusively proven that injecting a foreign substance into the disk and perforating the annulus does not damage an otherwise normal disk. All these objections would be acceptable if the test provided unequivocal information, *which it does not*.

Electromyography (EMG) is an objective test that may validate nerve root impairment and aid in localizing the root level. When there is doubt that the site of nerve root impairment is at the neck level, the brachial plexus, or somewhat distally in the extremity, the EMG may assist. The EMG is a valuable diagnostic aid when positive, and when negative may serve to improve the prognosis. The malingerer who feigns total paralysis is frequently revealed by a normal EMG. Unfortunately, the EMG enjoys unjustified medical-legal prominence. It must be remembered that nerve damage does not manifest positive EMG changes for the first three weeks, so a negative EMG before that time does not indicate absence of nerve damage. EMG evidence of

54

demyelinization may also have been present before an alleged injury as the result of an infectious disease, inflammatory condition, or previous injury.

In summary, the diagnosis of neck pain with or without referred pain relies upon a carefully taken history and a carefully interpreted physical examination. Adjunctive tests perform a confirmatory function at best and should always be interpreted in that light.

REFERENCES

1. Holdsworth, F. W.: Fractures, dislocation and fracture dislocations of the spine. J. Bone Joint Surg. 45-B:6–20, 1963.
2. McRae, D. L.: Asymptomatic intervertebral disc protrusions. Acta Radiol. 46:9–27, 1956.
3. Lindblom, K.: Diagnostic puncture of intervertebral disks in sciatica. Acta Orthop. Scand. 17:231–9, 1948.
4. Sneider, S. E., Winslow, O. P., Jr., and Pryor, T. H.: Cervical diskography: Is it relevant? J.A.M.A. 185:163–5, 1963.
5. Smith, G. W.: Normal cervical diskogram; with clinical observations. Am. J. Roentg. 81:1006–10, 1959.
6. Rabinovitch, R.: Diseases of intervertebral disk and its surrounding tissues. Springfield, Ill., Charles C Thomas, 1961.

BIBLIOGRAPHY

Brain, R.: Spondylosis, the known and the unknown. Lancet 1:687–93, 1954.
Cloward, R. B.: Lesions of the intervertebral disk and their treatment by interbody fusion method. Clin. Orthop. 27:51–77, 1963.
Gordon, E. E.: Natural history of the intervertebral disc. Arch. Phys. Med. Rehabil. 42:750–63, 1961.
Sandler, B.: Cervical spondylosis as a cause of spinal cord pathology. Arch. Phys. Med. Rehabil. 42:650–60, 1961.
White, J. C. and Sweet, W. H.: Pain: Its mechanisms and neurosurgical control. Springfield, Ill., Charles C Thomas, 1955.

CHAPTER 4

Cervical Disk Disease as a Factor in Pain and Disability

Pain originating in the neck but felt in the shoulder, arm, hand, or neck most frequently results from irritation of the cervical nerve roots in the region of the intervertebral foramina. The mechanism of pain originating in the neck region can broadly be considered as *resulting from encroachment of space or a faulty movement or position.*

The size and shape of the foramina of the functional units largely depend upon the integrity of the intervertebral disks (see Fig. 1). Normal disk tissue in the static spine maintains separation of the vertebral bodies and the posterior joints. The foramen is intact. Neck movement causes gliding movement of one vertebra upon another, which distorts the disk. The normal disk permits physiological distortion and recovery without permitting excessive distortion of the intervertebral or spinal canal openings. The neck ligaments help maintain the shape of the disks while preventing excessive distortion.

A defect in the disk can influence the relationship of the vertebral components and alter the size and shape of the foramina in both the static and the kinetic state.[1] The contents of the foramina, the nerves and blood vessels, are exposed to irritation from pressure, traction, angulation, and inflammation; thus encroachment into the foramen causes pain and dysfunction.

NATURE AND MECHANISM OF RADICULAR PAIN

There is some controversy that pain in the neck, arm, and shoulder may be due primarily to disk pathology rather than due to compression of nerve roots or their contiguous tissues.[2,3] This idea is entertained even though the disk has no confirmed nerve supply.

Symptoms attributed to the disk per se are claimed to occur weeks or months before there is any neurological evidence of root entrapment. Pain, after a neck injury, was located in the region of the scapula with local tenderness and palpable muscle spasm in that region and with relief afforded by infiltration of Novocain.[2, 3] The interscapular painful area was found to show hyperirritability on EMG examination[2-4] but no evidence of nerve damage.

The muscles of this interscapular area receive their nerve supply as follows:

levator scapula muscles	C_3–C_4
rhomboid muscles	C_5
supraspinatus and infraspinatus	C_5–C_6
latissimus dorsi muscles	C_6–C_7

The skin dermatome area over this area is supplied by T_7.

The interscapular pain was concluded, therefore, to be muscular pain of a reflex nature rather than compression of a *single* nerve root, either motor or sensory.

Scapular pain induced by stimulating the cervical disk is similar in character to pain which Frykholm[5] elicited when he irritated the ventral (motor) nerve roots intradurally. This pain was found to be "more deeply situated and referred to the proximal part of the limb and shoulder girdle . . . (that were) tender to pressure." This sensation was different from the pain elicited by stimulation of the sensory nerve roots.

Diskography, a technique of injecting dye into the nucleus of the cervical disk, has verified (1) entrance of dye specifically into the nucleus of a *specific* disk, (2) the normality or abnormality of that specific disk by visualization on X-rays, (3) symptoms resulting from injection of dye into that disk can be specified by the patient, and (4) the exact area of the disk irritated can be verified and related to the specific pain pattern elicited.[6]

Differentiation of diskogenic pain from neurogenic pain was suggested by diskography.[6] In the performance of the diskography, merely touching the anterior surface of the disk with the needle caused pain in the "shoulder blade" or the interscapular region. This pain could be abolished by injection, through the diskogram needle, of a small amount of an anesthetic agent.

Performance of diskography revealed various patterns of scapular pain depending upon the site and direction of disk nuclear herniation (Fig. 41). The logical conclusion is that pain referred from the disk due to herniation *within* the disk is located in the scapular-interscapular area of referral. It has vague localization value in that the superior disks refer to a superior level and lower diskogenic levels are referred more caudally.

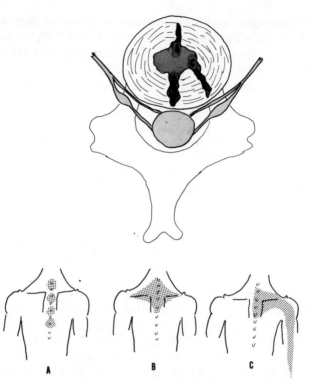

FIGURE 41. Referral sites of pain elicited by intranuclear diskograms. *A,* Irritation of the anterior portion of the disk refers pain to the interscapular midline. *B,* Posterior nucleus protrusion refers pain as depicted. *C,* Posterior lateral protrusion into the region of the intervertebral foramen causes interscapular pain *plus* arm radicular pain in the distribution of the nerve root dermatome.

Neurogenic pain from disk herniation is only felt when the protrusion encroaches upon the nerve roots within the foraminal gutter. This more distal radiation is also accompanied by shoulder and interscapular pain from irritation into the posterior primary division of the nerve roots.

Radicular pain varies from a deep, aching pain to a sharp pain superimposed on a dull, aching background. *It is often common for radicular pain to be felt proximally and paresthesia or a sensation of numbness to be felt distally.*

Pain has been classified as *neuralgic* or *myalgic,* depending upon the specific component of the nerve root involved. Irritation of the *sensory* portion of the nerve root causes *neuralgic* pain, and *myalgic* pain is caused by irritation of the ventral motor nerve root. Experimentally, stimulation of the dorsal root elicits "lightning" or "electric-shocklike" pain[7] felt maximally at the periphery of the extremity. The area of pain sensation conforms to a specific skin area known as a dermatome. Stimulation of the ventral motor root causes pain proximally in the shoulder, axilla, and upper arm described as a deep, "boring," unpleasant sensation. This pain is vague and generally localized in deep tissues such as muscles, tendons, and fascial planes. These areas are termed sclerotomic regions.

The ventral roots are essentially motor in function, and the exact mechanism of ventral root pain is unknown. Such experimentally induced ventral root pain appears to contradict the Bell-Magendie Law, but is postulated to be based on antidromic impulses and possible only in the presence of an intact dorsal root. The sensory topography of ventral-root-referred pain conforms in part to the muscle groups innervated by the roots and thus refer pain in a myotomic area.

The area to which pain is referred and in which numbness and tingling is felt has proximal localization at certain levels in the cervical cord. Certain muscle groups are innervated by motor roots also having localization in the cervical cord. In spite of the specificity of the sensory and motor roots in their dermatomic and myotomic distribution, there is too much overlapping and vagueness of localization of the symptoms and findings to designate specifically *one root* at *one level*.

The specific type of nerve irritation causing pain is not fully understood. Pressure alone on a nerve is not considered to cause pain. Nerves exposed to pressures of 2000 to 7000 lb per sq in showed no defect in nerve conduction.[8] Ischemia blocks impulse conduction but this block is reversible.[9]

As stated in Chapter 1, and shown in Figures 29 and 30, neck flexion causes upward movement of the nerves within the spinal canal[10] but there is no movement of the extradural root pouches.[10, 11] The roots[10, 12, 13] are firmly fixed at the outer rim of the intervertebral foramen but there is considerable movement up and down in the medial (inner) aspect of the intervertebral foramina. This movement of the intrathecal (intraspinal) roots pivots upon their point of fixation at the outer aspect of the intervertebral foramen. With the head extended the roots *ascend* into the foramen, while in the flexed position the roots *descend* (Fig. 42). They are more *tense* when descended, i.e., in the flexed position of the neck. Movement of the roots (ascending and descending) increases after 25 years of age and remains constant at age 40. This is based probably on the fact that the dural sac remains at a constant length whereas the spine shortens due to disk degeneration.

The dural sac unfolds and actually stretches during neck flexion. The dural sac tenses and literally constricts the extraneural space. This is considered to cause ischemia when the dural sac becomes taut. The dentate ligaments transmit forces from the dural sac to the cord (not the roots).[11] As the neck flexes, the dural sac is stretched drawing

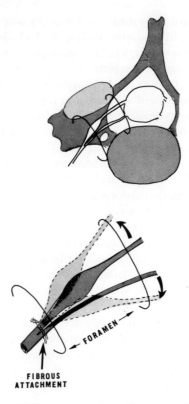

FIGURE 42. Movement of nerve roots about their point of attachment. The nerve roots are anchored at the outer area of the formen. As the intradural nerves move, cranially during flexion and caudally during neck extension, the roots angle about their fibrous attachment (point of fixation). This explains increased nerve tension during these movements.

the dentate ligaments apart. They thus pull the dural sac laterally and narrow the anterior-posterior width thus compressing only the cord.

The degree of lordosis and kyphosis (flexion) is stated to be "range of motion." This can be in part determined by lateral X-rays taken in flexion and extension. Unfortunately, neck pain in cervical spondylosis limits the reliability of these X-rays.

"Root pain" (spondylotic radiculopathy) is usually considered to be caused by compression of the extradural root passing through the foramen.[14, 15] On neck extension, the foraminal size decreases[11, 15] and it is considered that pressure upon the entrapped roots cause the pain. It is difficult to use this explanation when the foramina are *not* small on X-ray or when there is ankylosis of the zygapophyseal joints permitting no movement. Bradshaw[17] noted poor surgical results when there were no "structural" abnormalities.

Stretching of the extrathecal root is probably more the cause than a compression. An osteophyte either within the foramen or a posterior lateral vertebral space can elongate the dural sac and place it under tension.

Flexion (kyphosis) causes the roots to descend and become more taut. Extension causes the roots to ascend and the foramen to narrow. Either can cause root ischemia. The clinical reproduction of root pain helps determine the cause of pain which treatment must alter.

The effect upon the nerve root from narrowing of the intervertebral foramen from disk degeneration and zygapophyseal (facet) degeneration causes a lesion of the posterior nerve root. The lesion occurs particularly at its junction with the dorsal root ganglion or to the root ganglion itself (see Fig. 32). The anterior (motor) nerve roots are rarely damaged.[18]

Irritation by compression of the nerve root (ganglion) results in diffuse increase of the fibrous tissue of the endoneurium which encircles the neuron. With increasing fibrous reaction, the nerve undergoes demyelination with simultaneous increase of perineural collagen.[19, 20]

The most severely damaged nerve roots are C_6 and C_7 causing pain and paresthesia down the radial aspect of the arm into the hand and fingers. This is true because at this midcervical region there is the greatest mobility, greatest angulation, and the greatest amount of disk degeneration[21] (see discussion in Chapter 1).

Flexion of the neck thus further deforms the nerve root and distorts it. Extension of the neck reduces the diameter of the foramen that is already diminished by the disk degeneration, osteophyte formation, and the apophysial joint arthritic changes.

It must be remembered that there is a discrepancy between the radiological changes in the cervical spine and the degree and *distribution* of neurological symptoms. This discrepancy is due to (1) soft tissue abnormality not seen on X-rays, (2) excessive or limited movement of the cervical spine, (3) variation in nerve root formation, (4) shortening of the spinal canal due to aging and disk degeneration causing a change in nerve root alignment (see Fig. 30) and angulation, (5) change in the contour of the cervical spine, i.e., acute kyphotic angulation in the normally lordotic curved spine due to segmental disk degeneration caused by injury, and (6) lateral scoliosis due to asymmetric disk degeneration causing unilateral intervertebral foraminal closure on the concave side. There may also be a discrepancy of the size of the nerve roots as compared with the size of the foraminal opening.

Change (movement) is essential for an irritant upon a nerve to cause pain; therefore if *pressure does not change, pain does not result* or does not persist. If this concept of pain causation is correct, a basic tenet of treatment is specified.

61

Traction upon a nerve is considered a pain-producing stimulus. The mechanism is thought to be that stretching the nerve stretches the dural sheath of the nerve and thereby impairs its blood supply, the ischemia of the nerve causing the pain.

An interesting concept of pain production has been depicted in Figure 23. This concept is that pain does not result from nerve root pressure or irritation, but rather that irritation of the nerve root causes a reflex muscle spasm, and the muscle spasm becomes the site of pain, the sensation of which returns to the cord by the sensory pathways.[22]

Regardless of the exact mechanism of pain production, it is evident that (1) nerve irritation must occur, (2) if pressure is an irritant, it must be acute and intermittent, and (3) the nerve must be entrapped so as to be unable to avoid fully the impact of the irritant. The concept of neck pain because of inadequate space or faulty movement applies.

Unchanging pressure upon a nerve results in impaired nerve function, such as (1) partial loss of sensory function (hypesthesia), (2) complete loss of sensory transmission (anesthesia), and (3) motor impairment (weakness, paralysis, reflex changes and their objective demonstration such as atrophy). Pain resulting from pressure and movement and functional loss resulting from persistent movement both imply merely degrees of the same mechanism.

CERVICAL DISK

The cervical disk plays a vital role in many conditions of the neck that cause local pain or referred pain in the upper extremities. In its function as a "joint" between two vertebrae composing the anterior portion of the functional unit the cervical disk permits movement and simultaneously helps keep the foramina apart, and it maintains proper alignment so that the spinal canal and the vertebral artery foramina retain their integrity. By maintaining the separation of the vertebrae anteriorly, the disks maintain the proper relationship of the articulations posteriorly.

Nerve root compression from disk herniation is infrequent. To contact the nerve, the disk must herniate into the intervertebral foramen and thus protrude in a dorsolateral direction. This direction of disk herniation is prevented or at least minimized by the interposition of the joints of von Luschka, which are bony elevations from the dorsolateral portions of the vertebral bodies forming a wall between the annulus of the disk and the coursing nerve root through the foramen.

The nerve is further protected from bulging of the disk by the posterior longitudinal ligament completely enclosing the disk posteriorly with a firm, double layered ligament. This arrangement differs from the lumbar area where the posterior longitudinal ligament (in the lower lumbar area) is incomplete, thin, and single layered and can permit herniation of the disk through the lateral areas unprotected by the ligament (Fig. 43).

The nucleus of the disk in the cervical region is located anteriorly in the wide portion of the disk space. Mechanically this location prevents movement backward into a narrower area. To move posteriorly would require compression of the nucleus, an action that is resisted by the viscosity of the nuclear gel.

The annulus fibrosus is much thicker and denser in the posterior lateral portion of the disk, thus more resistant to distension in this area. Herniation of the disk in the dorsolateral direction necessary to permit nerve contact within the foraminal gutter is minimized because (1) the nerve roots emerge from the cord opposite the vertebral bodies, with the uppermost fibers of the root barely in contact with the inferior margin of the above disk and the lower fibers nowhere near the next lower disk (see Fig. 26), (2) more dorsolaterally in its course into and through the foraminal canal the bony protrusion (so-called joint of von Luschka) separates the nerve from the annulus of the disk,

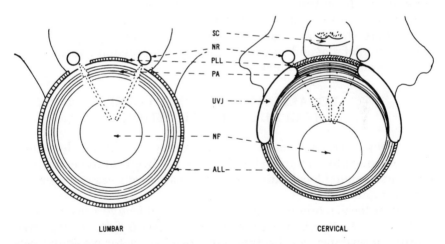

LUMBAR

CERVICAL

FIGURE 43. Comparison of lumbar and cervical disk containers. The *lumbar* region has an incomplete posterior longitudinal ligament, *PLL*, a thin layer posteriorly of the annulus fibrosus, *PA*, and thus a relatively exposed nerve root, *NR*. Arrows show the routes by which herniation of the nucleus can approach the nerve roots. The nucleus pulposus, *NP*, is centrally located. The *cervical* region has a posterior longitudinal ligament, *PLL*, spanning the entire posterior portion of the vertebral body, a double layered ligament. The posterior portion of the annulus, *PA*, is broader and firmer. The nerve root, *NR*, is partially protected by the interposed uncovertebral joints of von Luschka, *UVJ*, and the anterior position of the nucleus, *NP*, places it far from the nerve roots and the spinal cord. All these factors protect the nerve roots and the spinal cord, *SP*, from the protruding disk material.

(3) the entire posterior portion of the annulus is reinforced by a strong, double layered, posterior longitudinal ligament, (4) the very shape of the disk (wide anteriorly and narrow posteriorly) tends to keep the nucleus in the wider anterior portion, and last, (5) the annulus is broader and firmer in its posterior region, which reinforces the disk where it is closest to the nerve root. All these factors do not favor herniation of disk material as a common source of nerve root pressure. The literature is permeated with claims ranging from complete denials that disk herniation causes nerve root pressure to claims that it is the commonest cause of radiculopathy. If disk protrusion posteriorly were common, herniation would be a common cause of spinal cord compression, but it is not.

Disk herniations are further classified into *soft* disks and *hard* disks depending upon what tissue portion of the disk protrudes.[23] The *soft* variety consists mostly of nuclear material; the *hard* type is mostly annular fibroelastic tissue[14] that may or may not be partially calcified. The *hard* disk protrusion is considered most prevalent. When a *hard* disk protrusion is found in the posterolateral region, it is frequently impossible to differentiate the bulging mass between calcified disk material and hypertrophied bony uncovertebral joint material.[24]

Six possible directions of disk herniation are postulated. These directions are shown in Figure 44, and the possible nerve root, cord, combination of root and cord, and vascular compression effect of each type of protrusion is evident.

LOCALIZATION OF ROOT LEVEL BY CLINICAL EXAMINATION

Accuracy of cervical root localization other than by myelography, electromyography, or surgical exploration has been controversial over the years. General localization of approximate levels has been reasonably accurate.

Clinical localization is determined by (1) subjective sensory localization by area in which pain or hyperesthesia is felt, (2) objective sensory dermatomal localization, (3) subjective motor weakness verified by (4) objective muscle testing (myotome) and (5) deep tendon reflex determination.

As most lesions involve roots C_5, C_6, C_7, or C_8, the accuracy of localization is enhanced. Left-sided versus right-sided is evident.

Pain localization[25] is vague and usually nonlocalizing. Pain in the neck, shoulder, scapula, or interscapular area is *nonlocalizing* in regard to specifying a specific root level or at best localizes two root levels.

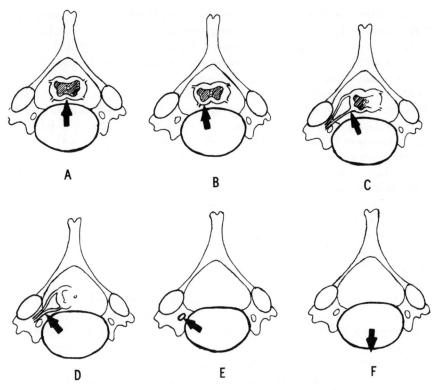

FIGURE 44. Possible results from direction of disk herniation.

A = Dorsomedial herniation may cause bilateral cord compression.
B = Paramedial herniation: unilateral cord compression.
C = Dorsolateral protrusion: unilateral cord and nerve root compression.
D = Intraforaminal protrusion: radicle nerve root compression.
E = Lateral protrusion: vertebral artery and nerve compression.
F = Ventral protrusion causes no nerve root, cord, or vertebral artery compression.

Pain in the upper arm is not specific. Reference to the posterior aspect of the arm is most often C_7 whereas medial, anterior, or lateral localization can be C_6, C_7, or both.

Localization by pain in the forearm is also limited as to specifying one root level. Forearm pain usually specifies C_6 or C_7 but is not specific for one root.

Pain or paresthesia in the hand is more accurate. Paresthesia of the thumb (and only the thumb) usually indicates compression of C_6. If the thumb *and* the next finger or fingers are hyperesthetic, localization of *one* root is less accurate. Paresthesia of the index finger and middle finger (with or without thumb or ring finger) is most often C_7. Paresthesia of the ulnar fingers (ring and little fingers) is usually C_8.

Subjective weakness[26] is of limited localizing value. Weakness of the shoulder (arm elevation) tends to incriminate C_5 and weakness of the hand and fingers C_8.

Objective weakness[27] by muscle testing is a more specific test for localizing root level. In fact a *careful muscle test is probably the most accurate portion of an examination to specify a specific root level.*

C_5 weakness is best located by deltoid (arm abduction) and supraspinatus-infraspinatus (external arm rotation) testing.

C_6 is best tested by weakness of the brachialis (elbow flexion with forearm in neutral position from pronation and supination) and weakness of the biceps (forearm supination).

C_7 is best localized by finding weakness of the triceps (elbow extensors) but can be confirmed by finding weakness of the flexor carpi ulnaris and radialis, pronator teres (pronation of the wrist and forearm) and extensor pollicis longus (extension of the distal phalanx of the thumb).

All the muscle tests must be performed to specifically localize a muscle action with other actions being minimized. The deltoid can be examined with the patient standing. The biceps is best tested with the patient seated. The triceps and external rotators of the upper arm are best tested with the patient supine.

The triceps can be easily tested by resisting extension of the arm moving toward the ceiling. This can be tested by manual resistance or by the use of graded dumbbells (Fig. 45). Endurance testing may

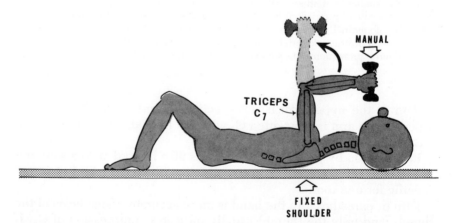

FIGURE 45. Muscle examination of triceps (C_7). With patient supine and arm held vertically, the triceps can more easily be tested for strength and for endurance. In this position the scapular muscles are fixed, allowing the triceps to be isolated (C_7). Fatigue may indicate a C_7 lesion when a single effort fails to reveal weakness.

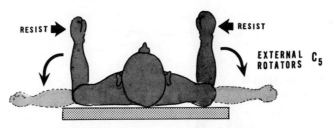

FIGURE 46. External rotator testing to test the supraspinatus and infraspinatus muscles and determine integrity of C_5 root. The patient is best placed in the supine position with arms held at the side. Resisting the forearm as patient attempts external rotation facilitates this muscle examination.

reveal weakness when one contraction does not reveal significant or discernible weakness. Fatigue or inability after 5 to 15 contractions will indicate a root level involvement. In the case of the triceps, a C_7 root involvement.

With the patient in the supine position the external rotators can be easily tested. With the elbows held at the side, moving the hands outward toward the table can easily be resisted and tested (Fig. 46).

Testing the intrinsics of the fingers (abduction and adduction) tests root C_8.

Objective sensory testing[28] must be performed to test hypalgesia and hypasthesia. The former is best tested by pin prick or pin scratch and the latter tested by sensation of cotton or cloth. The levels found usually conform to the subjective dermatomal patterns.[25]

Localization by testing deep tendon reflexes has value *if* the reflex is properly tested. The triceps jerk is diminished in a C_7 root involvement but may also be diminished in a lesion of C_8; thus finding a diminished triceps reflex *per se is not localizing.* The brachioradialis reflex may be diminished in C_7 lesions but its absence usually indicates a C_6 root level lesion.

Brachioradialis Reflex

This reflex initiates a brisk stretching and response of the brachioradialis muscle. This muscle originates from the lateral border of the humerus above the epicondyle and inserts on the lateral side of the lower end of the radius. It is essentially a flexor of the elbow and has some limited ability to pronate (from a supinated position) or to supinate the wrist (from a pronated position).

The brachioradialis reflex is performed with the forearm in a neutral midposition of pronation and supination of the flexed elbow (Fig. 47).

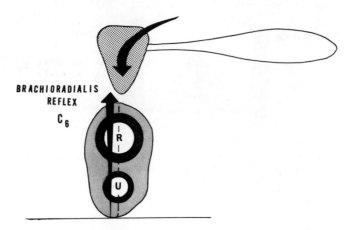

BRACHIORADIALIS
REFLEX
C$_6$

FIGURE 47. Brachioradialis reflex. With the forearm gently supported and neutral between pronation and supination, a gentle tap on the distal radius or the styloid (attachment of the brachioradialis muscle) will cause reflex flexion of the elbow. The fingers may also flex but are *not* a portion of the B.R. reflex. With finger flexion and *no* elbow flexion, this "reversal" implies a C$_6$ lesion.

The reflex is mediated via the C$_6$ root. In a lesion of this root, attempting to elicit the reflex will possibly cause flexion of the fingers but *no elbow flexion*. This finding is termed inversion of the radial reflex.[29]

Pronator Reflex

Tapping the lower portion of the radius causes a reflex pronation—the pronator reflex (Fig. 48). This reflex is mediated through the pronator teres and pronator quadratus muscles, both of C$_7$ (some C$_6$ and C$_8$ but principally C$_7$) innervation. The technique must be gentle and subtle, i.e., the reflex hammer must be swung gently to stretch the pronator muscles and not overflow to other confusing muscle contractions.

The position of the forearm is important. It must rest on its ulnar side in a neutral position (see Fig. 48) or slightly pronated. If the position of the forearm is varied or the tap misdirected, other muscles may be stimulated and a different reflex elicited (such as the brachioradialis, biceps, or finger flexor), thus implicating a different root level.

The pronator reflex is especially valuable in the early diagnosis of upper motor neuron lesions (pyramidal) thus alerting the examiner to the possibility of cervical myelopathy. The reflex may be hyperactive and clonus may also be noted.

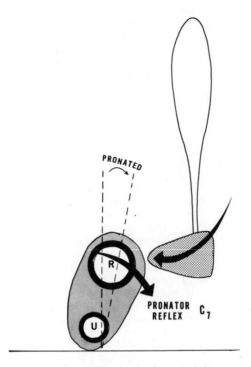

FIGURE 48. Pronator reflex. With the forearm slightly pronated (10–15°) and lightly supported, the reflex hammer is swung gently to tap the radial styloid on the volar surface. This reflexly stretches the pronator teres and causes the forearm to pronate. This reflex is mediated via the C_7 root.

Summary

The following characteristics localize specific root levels:

Root	Referred Pain	Paresthesia	Weakness	Reflex
C_5	shoulder and upper arm	none in digit	shoulder	biceps
C_6*	radial aspect forearm	thumb	biceps brachioradialis wrist extensor	biceps
C_7†	dorsal aspect forearm	index and middle fingers	triceps	triceps
C_8††	ulnar aspect forearm	ring and little fingers	finger intrinsics	triceps

* Figure 49.
† Figure 50.
†† Figure 51.

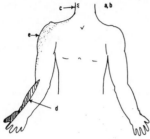

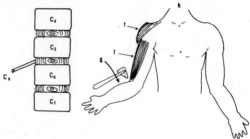

FIGURE 49. Sixth cervical nerve root irritation.

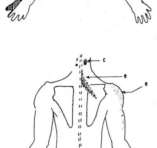

a = Neck rigidity. Limited extension and rotation to the right.
b = Pain and paresthesia aggravated by coughing and sneezing.
c = Tenderness over exit of C_6 nerve root.
d = Paresthesia and hypasthesia of thumb and some of index finger (from history and physical examination).
e = Subjective pain and tenderness over deltoid and rhomboid muscle area.
f = Weakness of deltoid and biceps muscles.
g = Depressed biceps jerk.
h = X-rays equivocal.

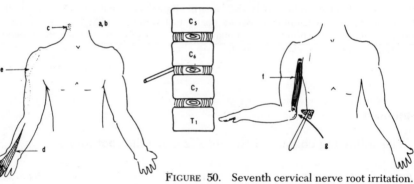

FIGURE 50. Seventh cervical nerve root irritation.

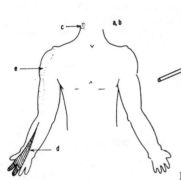

a = Neck rigidity. Limited extension and rotation to the involved side.
b = Pain and paresthesia aggravated by coughing and sneezing.
c = Tenderness over exit of C_7.
d = Paresthesia and hypasthesia of index and middle finger.
e = Subjective deep pain and tenderness of dorsolateral upper arm and superiormedial angle of scapula.
f = Weakness of triceps (also possibly biceps).
g = Depressed triceps jerk.

70

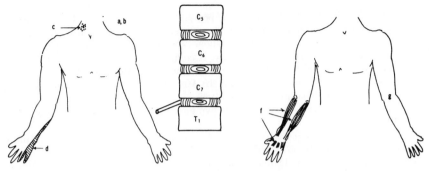

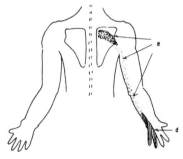

FIGURE 51.   Eighth cervical nerve root irritation.

a = Neck rigidity. Limited extension and rotation to the involved side.
b = Pain and paresthesia aggravated by coughing and sneezing.
c = Tenderness over exit of C_8.
d = Paresthesia and hypasthesia of inner forearm and little finger.
e = Subjective deep pain and tenderness from scapula down *inner* side of upper arm, inner forearm, to little finger.
f = Weakness of hand muscles.
g = No reflex changes.

It can be noted that most muscles, most reflexes, and the sensory dermatomal patterns have multiple root innervation, thus it cannot be stated that specific findings locate a single root. Rather, it is necessary to do numerous reflex examinations, many careful muscle examinations, and careful sensory dermatomal examination by light touch and pin scratch *THEN*, by deduction from compiling all findings, determine the most logical nerve root. Subsequent electromyography utilizing the same deductive analysis of numerous muscle samplings will confirm the clinical impression.

REFERENCES

1. Gordon, E. E.: Natural history of the intervertebral disc. Arch. Phys. Med. Rehabil. 42:750–63, 1961.
2. Elliott, F. A. and Kremer, M.: Brachial pain from herniation of cervical intervertebral disk. Lancet 1:4–8, 1944.
3. Michelson, J. J. and Mixter, W. J.: Pain and disability of shoulder and arm due to herniation of the nucleus pulposus of cervical intervertebral disks. N. Engl. J. Med. 231:279–87, 1944.
4. Wedell, G., Feinstein, B., and Pattle, A.: The clinical application of electromyography. Lancet 1:236–38, 1945.

5. Frykholm, R.: Deformities of dural pouches and structures of dural sheaths in cervical region producing nerve root compression: Contribution to etiology and operative treatment of brachial neuralgia. J. Neurosurg. 4:403–13, 1947.
6. Cloward, R. B.: Cervical diskography: A contribution to the etiology and mechanism of neck, shoulder and arm pain. Ann. Surg. 150:1052–64, 1959.
7. White, J. C. and Sweet, W. H.: Pain: Its Mechanisms and Neurosurgical Control. Springfield, Ill., Charles C Thomas, 1955.
8. Grundfest, H.: Cold Spring Harbor Symposium on Quantitative Biology. 4:179, 1936.
9. Causey, G.: Functional importance of blood supply of peripheral nerves. Ann. R. Coll. Surg. Engl. 16:367, 1955.
10. Reed, J. D.: Effects of flexion-extension movements of the head and spine upon the spinal cord and nerve roots. J. Neurol. Neurosurg. Psychiat. 23:214–21, 1960.
11. Adams, C. B. T. and Logue, V.: Studies in cervical spondylotic myelopathy I. Movement of the cervical roots, dura and cord, and their relation to the course of the extradural roots. Brain. 94:557–68, 1971.
12. Brieg, A.: Biomechanics of the Central Nervous System. Stockholm, Almquist and Wiksell, 1960.
13. Hadley, L. A.: The Spine: Anatomico-Radiographic Studies, Development and the Cervical Region. Springfield, Ill., Charles C Thomas, 1956.
14. Frykholm, R.: Cervical nerve root compression resulting from disc degeneration and root-sleeve fibrosis: A clinical investigation. Acta Chir. Scand. Supp. 160, 1951.
15. Waltz, T. A.: Physical factors in the production of myelopathy of cervical spondylosis. Brain 90:395–404, 1967.
16. Pallis, C., Jones, A. M., and Spillane, J. D.: Cervical spondylosis. Brain 77:274–89, 1954.
17. Bradshaw, P.: Some aspects of cervical spondylosis. Quart. J. Med. 26:177–208, 1957.
18. Holt, S. and Yates, P. O.: Cervical spondylosis and nerve root lesions. J. Bone Joint Surg. 48A:407–23, 1966.
19. Causey, G.: Electron Microscopy. Edinburgh and London, Livingston, p. 202, 1962.
20. Barton, A. A.: An electron microscopic study of degeneration and regeneration of nerve. Brain 85:799, 1962.
21. Turner, E. L. and Oppenheimer, A.: A common lesion of the cervical spine responsible for segmental neuritis. Ann. Intern. Med. 10:427, 1936.
22. Cloward, R. B.: Lesions of the intervertebral disk and their treatment by interbody fusion method. Clin. Orthop. 27:51–77, 1963.
23. Brain, R.: Spondylosis, the known and the unknown. Lancet 1:687–93, 1954.
24. Sandler, B.: Cervical spondylosis as a cause of spinal cord pathology. Arch. Phys. Med. Rehabil. 42:650–60, 1961.
25. Steindler, A.: The cervical pain syndrome. In Instructional Course Lectures, The American Academy of Orthopedic Surgeons, Vol. XIV. Ann Arbor, J. W. Edwards, 1957.
26. Armstrong, J. R.: Lumbar Disc Lesions. Edinburgh and London, Livingston, 1952.
27. Fielding, J. W.: Cineroentgenography of the normal cervical spine. J. Bone Joint Surg. 39-A:1280–1, 1957.
28. Jackson, R.: The Cervical Syndrome, 2nd ed. Springfield, Ill., Charles C Thomas, 1958.
29. Walsche, F. M. R. and Ross, J.: The clinical picture of minor cord lesions in association with injuries of the cervical spine. Brain 59:277, 1936.

CHAPTER 5

Subluxations of the Cervical Spine Including the "Whiplash" Syndrome

"Whiplash" of the neck is a controversial term enjoying no unanimity of understanding and no acceptance of definition. Symptoms attributed to this syndrome are vaguely described, the etiology is dramatically explained, the mechanisms of injury are poorly understood, and the treatment is empirical at best. In this state of total confusion and ignorance the injured have been neglected, mistreated, and even accused of deception, while many uninjured complainers have been exhorbitantly and unjustifiably rewarded.[1]

Medical literature swings like a pendulum from complete denial of any such entity to verification and acceptance of every ramification of the injury. Such a denial is evident in a medical journal editorial,* and an outstanding medical authority has made a similar comment.† These comments, on the other hand, have been refuted by serious pathological-anatomical studies of the symptoms claimed and the mechanisms involved. Hopefully, a middle ground exists in this controversy.

A collision, when the offending car moves at a rate as slow as 7 miles per hour can cause severe tissue damage and injury.[2] Cord concussion causing temporary quadriplegia without loss of consciousness can only be explained by distortion of the cervical spine due to translatory forces. (Refer to "Syndrome of Acute Central Spinal Cord Injury" later in this chapter.)

---

* "The neck is not a whip. . . . This diagnosis is vague and thoroughly unscientific. . . . There is a tendency for this terminology to be employed . . . through lack of sufficient knowledge to make a specific diagnosis. . . . The term to the honest is merely a bulwark behind which ignorance skulks; to the dishonest a mirage with which to confuse and delude."—D. M. Bosworth: Editorial. J. Bone Joint Surg. 41-A:16, 1959.

† "In its pure form and when rightly diagnosed, the symptoms of 'whiplash' injury are those of cervical muscular spasm often complicated by neurosis,"—D. Munro: Treatment of fractures and dislocations of the cervical spine, complicated by cervical-cord and root injuries. N. Engl. J. Med. 264:573, 1961.

A much better medical term for this condition would undoubtedly aid greater understanding and acceptance. A term such as "whiplash," however, is deeply entrenched both medically and legally, and change will come slowly if at all.

Various words used to describe "whiplash" injury deserve definition and clarification. The word *strain* is defined as "injury resulting from overuse, improper use,"[3] *Sprain,* from the Latin *exprimere* (to press up), is defined as an "injury to a joint with possible rupture of some of the ligaments and tendons but without dislocation or fracture."[3] *Dislocation,* on the other hand, from the Latin *dis* (apart) and *locus* (place), is described as "a disarrangement of the normal relation of bones that enter into the formation of a joint: otherwise known as a *luxation.*"[3]

A paradox appears in correlating these definitions. It is difficult to visualize a *sprain* causing rupture of the ligaments of a joint without causing some derangement of the opposing joint surfaces, which by definition is a degree of luxation or *subluxation.* If a "whiplash" injury is considered a *severe sprain,* a *sub*luxation injury must be assumed.

Since the ligaments and capsular tissues of the neck normally permit neck movement to a point considered to be "just short of dislocation,"[4] to reach this point and exceed it slightly would conform to the definition of *sprain,* not merely a *strain;* and *subluxation* must have occurred. The controversy is not the denial of the manner of injury, but the question of *sprain* or *strain, subluxation* or *no subluxation.*

A better term than "whiplash" is desirable, also, to describe the method of injury. When a patient is injured in a rear-end collision or receives an injury with similar action, the term *deceleration* or *acceleration* would serve more accurately to describe the mechanics of the force, and *hyperflexion* or *hyperextension,* to describe the reaction to the force by the head and neck if the injury is sustained by the cervical spine. The extent of injury can then be further defined by *sprain* or *strain,* with or without subluxation, dislocation, or fracture as the case may be. Thus a person seated in a stopped car violently struck from behind so that he is moved forward and his head "snapped" back can be described as having sustained an acute cervical sprain due to an acute hyperextension reaction to a deceleration injury. A diagnostic label should state pathology when possible, anatomical site of injury, and method of tissue insult. What has happened is obviously of greater value than what the label is. Unfortunately, today terminology is tantamount to definition.

A rear-end collision intitates a sequence of events affecting the cervical spine, its joints, ligaments, and musculature. A similar sequence can be evoked in any injury causing *abrupt hyperextension* or *hyperflexion* of the neck.

The impact abruptly propels the body in a linear horizontal direction. Due to inertia, the head remains in its initial position then abruptly moves in the opposite direction. The movement of the head must be in the direction of flexion or extension of the cervical spine.

The abrupt movement of the neck occurs before the neck muscles can relax and permit this motion. Acting upon the unprepared muscles initiates an *acute stretch reflex*. In a rear-end impact the head moves abruptly backward causing acute hyperextension of the cerivcal spine causing an acute stretch reflex of the neck flexors (Fig. 52). A head-on collision would cause the opposite reaction with the stretch reflex being of the extensor muscles as the head proceeds forward and the neck acutely flexes.

Normally a muscle that contracts does so with physiological relaxation of the antagonistic muscles and no stretch reflex of the contracting muscles. This is mediated through neurological reflexes within the cord. The antagonist muscles are not subjected to any stretch reflex phenomenon or at most the stretch reflex is moderated and coordinated.[5, 6]

If the stretch is acute, abrupt, and overwhelming, the muscle fibrils sustain an injury. This injury is to the *intrafusal* fibers essentially and the *extrafusal* fibers if the force is appropriately severe (Fig. 53). This initiates a proportionately strong *stretch reflex* with a forceful muscu-

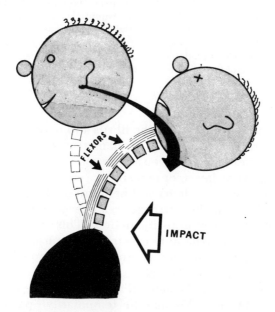

FIGURE 52. Neck flexor trauma from rear-end injury. Hyperextension causes an overstretch and inappropriate contraction of the neck flexors with residual flexor disability.

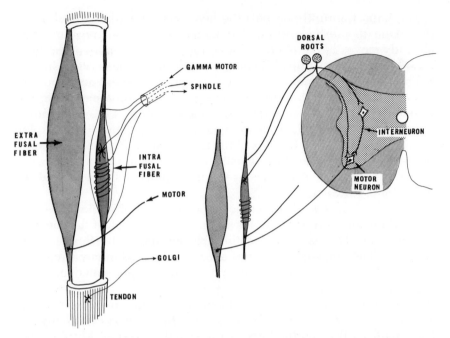

FIGURE 53. Muscle spindles. The contractile fibers are known as extrafusal fibers and are innervated by the motor neuron. The intrafusal fibers contain the spindles which end in annulospiral fibers and flower-spray endings. These fibers send impulses to the cord conveying stretch responses. In voluntary extrafusal contraction there is no stretch reflex. In an abrupt contraction of the extrafusal fibers, such as a tendon jerk, there is a reflex via the interneuron that stimulates the motor neuron. The tendon stretch is mediated through the Golgi tendon organ. The gamma motor fibers adjust the length and thus the response of the spindle system.

lar contraction. The injury is to the fibrils and not to the gross muscle bulk, thus there is usually no gross hemorrhage or edema. As major nerves are not initially involved, there may be no immediate pain, hyperesthesia, paresthesia, or paresis.

There *is* microscopic edema and hemorrhage combined with fibril injury. This edema and hemorrhage organize and form a "trigger" area or a resultant myofascial fibrositic nodule. This "traumatic fibrositis" remains as a focus of irritability causing more muscle irritability with muscular contracture, fibrous contracture, emotional reaction, and thus chronic pain and limitation.

Irritability or "spasm" is claimed and noted by patients and examiners. Initially the muscles may be temporarily "paralyzed" which accounts for so many patients the morning after an accident stating their inability to "lift their heads off the pillow."

76

When the muscles become overwhelmed and they are elongated past their physiological limits the fascial connective tissue, the tendons, the ligaments and the articular capsules are also overstretched and thus injured. As the joints are caused to exceed their physiological limits they essentially *sublux* causing all the periarticular tissue damage of a subluxation (Fig. 54). The magnitude of the reflex muscular contraction in response to the stretch is proportional to the abruptness and the strength of the stretching force.[7]

Flexion with the rebound in extension occurs in an acceleration injury. The person moving forward comes to a sudden stop. The lower body stops suddenly, and the heavy, suspended head proceeds forward by inertia to perform a flexion arc. If the impact is abrupt, unexpected, or overpowering to the extensor mechanism, *hyperflexion* results. Rebound occurs by extensor muscle reflex action and reverse inertia. The distorted arc of *re*-extension stresses the neck structures. Both *hyper*extension and *hyper*flexion result in *sprain* and *subluxation.*

Figure 55 shows the normal change, during physiological flexion, in the relationship of two vertebrae and the effect produced on the size and shape of the intervertebral foramina, and it shows the results of *hyperflexion.* The tissues bearing the brunt of hyperflexion are dia-

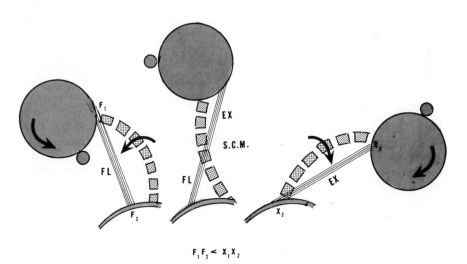

$$F_1 F_2 < X_1 X_2$$

FIGURE 54. Muscular reaction to "whiplash" injury. *Center,* Sternocleidomastoid muscle is extension (EX) to upper half of cervical spine and flexor (FL) to lower half. *Right,* Hyperextension, the S.C.M. is completely an extension and shorter than in neutral. *Left,* In flexion, the S.C.M. is completely flexor and shorter than neutral and hyperextension. This rapid movement overstretches muscle and causes a reflex inhibition and muscle strain.

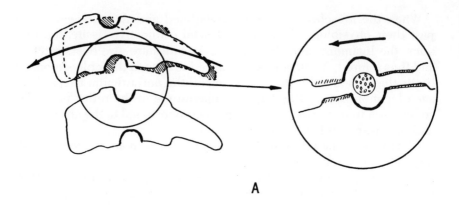

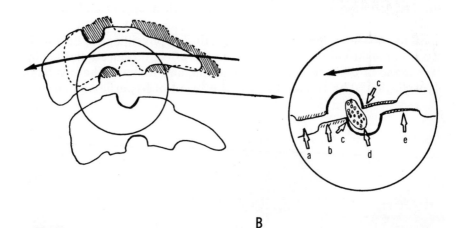

FIGURE 55. Mechanism of hyperflexion sprain injury to the neck. *A,* Normal forward gliding of the upper vertebra upon the lower and its effect upon the intervertebral foramen. *B, Hyper*flexion with disk distortion, *a,* foramen distortion, and nerve root impingement, *d,* anteriorly-inferiorly by the lower uncovertebral joint and superiorly-posteriorly by the upper articular facet, *c.* The articular facets are subluxed, *e.*

grammed in Figures 56 and 57. The converse of this flexion-hyper-flexion action on the functional unit (see Chapter 6, Fig. 74) shows the significance of pre-existing degenerative changes in potential damage from this type of injury.

Figure 58 shows possible injuries that can occur to the structures of the neck in hyperextension injury, and Figure 59 shows the effects of hyperflexion. The extent of injury to the tissues depends upon the force of impact, the exact position of the head at the moment of impact, the

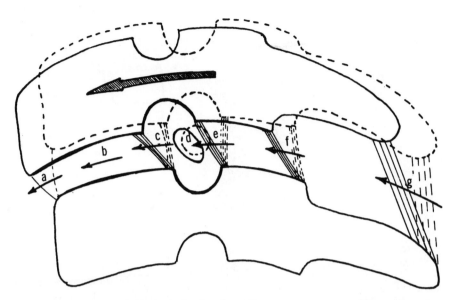

FIGURE 56. Tissues involved in hyperflexion sprain injury of the neck.

a = Anterior longitudinal ligament
b = Intervertebral disk
c = Posterior longitudinal ligament
d = Nerve root

e = Ligamentum flavum
f = Interspinous ligaments
g = Nuchal muscles

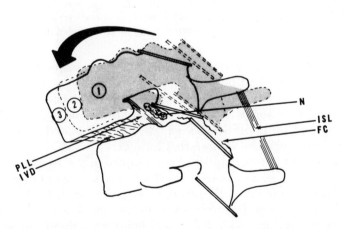

FIGURE 57. Hyperextension-hyperflexion injury. Normal physiologic flexion (1 to 2) is possible with no soft tissue damage. When motion is exceeded (3), the intervertebral disk (*IVD*) is pathologically deformed and the posterior longitudinal ligament (*PLL*) strained or torn; the nerve (*N*) is acutely entrapped; the facet capsule (*FC*) is torn or stretched; and the interspinous ligament (*ISL*) is damaged.

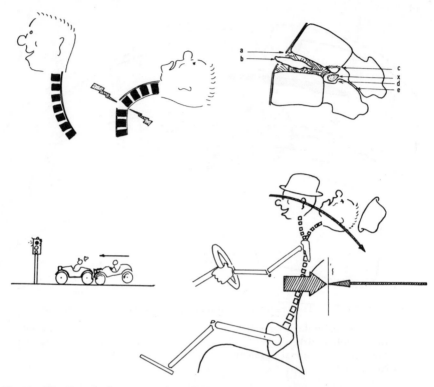

FIGURE 58. Rear-end impact with neck hyperextension sprain. When the patient is at a standstill, the impact from the rear causes an acute hyperextension movement of the neck. Possible injuries are *a*, anterior longitudinal tear; *b*, anterior herniation of intervertebral disk; *c*, chip fracture of vertebral body; *d*, facet encroachment into foramen; and *e*, acute facet impingement. The nerve root, *x*, can be impinged by this movement.

awareness of impending injury in order to "prepare" the musculature, and the normalcy of all the tissues of the neck.

Rarely does one direction of reaction to the jolt occur. Rebound is usual, so that flexion is followed by extension and vice versa. The tissues injured by hyperflexion may also be associated with injuries from the hyperextension phase that follows.

A concept of the mechanism of neck injury in the so-called "whiplash" injury has been advanced in which the movement of the body, rather than movement of the neck, causes the insult to the cervical spine. This theory is diagrammed in Figure 60. The head is considered to remain on the same horizontal level throughout the accident. The forward or backward movement of the body under the unmoving head causes an acute "shortening" of the neck; injury supposedly results from *compression* of the neck. These injuries are thus *compression-avulsion* injuries, not the flexion-extension traction injuries

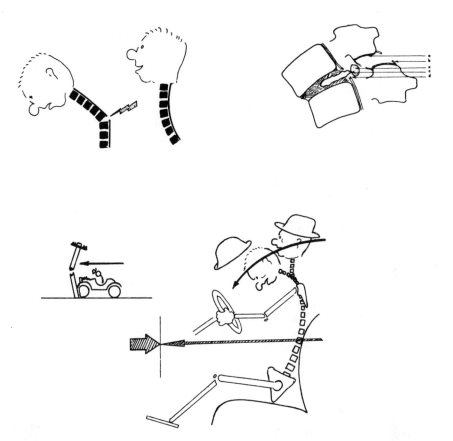

FIGURE 59. Flexion phase of acceleration injury to the neck (sprain). The body stops suddenly, but the neck continues due to continued momentum. The neck flexes and in fact may hyperflex. Possible injuries are *a*, an acute synovitis due to subluxation of the articular facets; *b*, capsular tear of articulation; *c*, posterior nuclear herniation; and *d*, posterior longitudinal ligamentous tear. All these may cause injury to the nerve root, *x*. The flexion phase of injury may be isolated, may follow as a "rebound" of an extension injury, or may be followed by a hyperextension phase (see Fig. 58).

depicted in Figures 58 and 59. Injury to the neck in this mechanism occurs as the exact vertical position of the head to the body is reached, not at either end of the accident. The *relaxed* position of the head and neck is considered more dangerous than the *taut*, alerted, *erect* position. Mathematically and geometrically, the neck is considered to *shorten* as much as an inch or more and to be under a compressive force of 500 to 600 pounds. Seatbelts are thought to place the person in the taut, erect position, thus minimizing the trauma to the neck in these accidents.

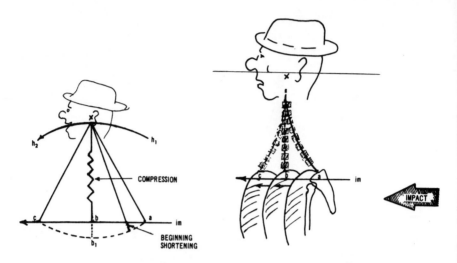

FIGURE 60. Compression theory of "whiplash" injury. The impact is taken by the body, which moves horizontally, *im*. The head does not move either up or down or forward or backward. The length of the neck at rest, *xa*, (before impact) shortens to length *xb* at the moment when the head is vertically above the body. At this midpoint the length of the neck should be xb_1; therefore, at this point there is compression. At the end of the impact movement, the neck regains its full length, *xc* (equal to *xa*). The diagram on the left shows the pathway of the neck when the mechanism is that of *neck movement upon the body*, h_1 to h_2 (see Figs. 55, 56 and 58). The length remains the same throughout the entire arc and at best causes *traction* upon the cervical spine.

This theory has been mathematically and geometrically refuted in that the head *does* rise above the horizontal plane during the impact, and it does so in a "loft" maneuver that involves extension or flexion in a torque direction (Fig. 61). The refutation advances a theory of the neck injury mechanism from acceleration or deceleration in which (1) "shortening" and compression of the neck does occur, (2) the relaxed neck at the moment of impact is more vulnerable, (3) the body does move in a horizontal direction under the neck, *but* (4) the head does move upward and transcribes an arc, or torque, about the C_1 and at C_7. The torque causes the damage in the midcervical region.

Studies performed in vitro on comparing compressive forces to distraction forces upon intervertebral disks revealed interesting results.[8] These studies were performed mostly upon lumbar disks but the conclusions may well apply to the cervical disks.

The following conclusions were reached (Fig. 62):

1. The nucleus is a viscous liquid with its shape maintained by the surrounding walls of the container: the vertebral end plates and the surrounding annular fibers.

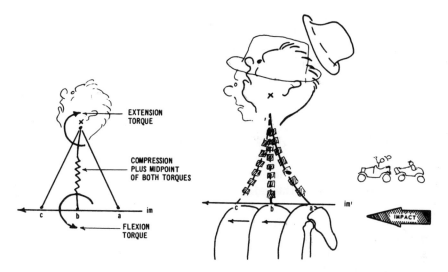

EXTENSION TORQUE

COMPRESSION PLUS MIDPOINT OF BOTH TORQUES

FLEXION TORQUE

FIGURE 61. Compression-plus-torque theory of cervical injury resulting from "whip-lash." The impact is taken by the body, which moves forward horizontally, *im*. Similar to Figure 60, there is compression of the cervical spine when reaching the vertical relation-ship of head directly over the body at the midpoint of the impact reaction. In contrast to Figure 60, the head is elevated and rotates (*torque*). The extension torque of C_1 and the flexion torque of C_7 place the avulsion stress in the midcervical region.

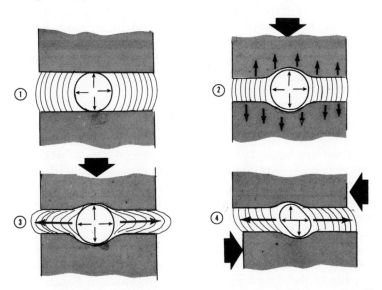

FIGURE 62. Mechanism of disk injuries. 1, Normal disk with form maintained by end plates and annulus. 2, Compression—the nucleus bulges into the end plates; the *large arrows* show blood being "squeezed" in the vertebral bodies. 3, Further compres-sion—or with dehydrated nucleus—pressure bulges the annulus out (*large arrows*). 4, Dehydrated nucleus permits excessive mobility of the unit.

83

2. Compression *does not* alter the shape of the nucleus. The compression bulges the vertebral end plates. The annulus bulges secondarily as the vertebral end plates approximate.
3. There is greater *annular bulge* when there is no nucleus pulposus.
4. Bulging of the end plate squeezes blood out of the cancellous bone.
5. Nuclear material *does not* cause a localized protrusion as the nucleus, being fluid, disperses evenly along the surfaces.
6. After loss of the nucleus there is abnormal mobility between the vertebral bodies and as there is no oozing of blood from the vertebral bodies, there is greater bulging of the annulus.

In a pure hyperflexion injury of a normal spine, before the posterior ligaments ruptured the vertebral bodies were crushed. In hyperextension injuries, the neural arch fractured before the anterior longitudinal ligament ruptured.

Only rotational forces or horizontal shearing forces caused disk damage. Therefore, it was concluded that cervical injuries of dislocation or fracture dislocation are undoubtedly due to rotational and/or shear forces rather than flexion-extension-compression caused disk damage.

These theories deny "whip" action of the head moving at the end of a flexible neck but confirm the concept of injury from flexion and extension with an avulsion stress. The theories stress movement of the body rather than primarily movement of the head as the mechanism, and *compression* rather than *traction*. The site of neck injury is the same and the tissue damage similar.

Protection from a seatbelt about the waist is difficult to accept in either of these theories or in one accepting principally neck movement. The taut, erect, alert position, looking directly forward, is the only unquestioned principle of safety. Cameron states, "At the present time there is no known mathematical premise which will explain all the forces of rear end collision. There are too many variables: among them *elasticity* of the neck and changes in the colliding masses."[9] In a medical approach to the problem, only the posture and elasticity of the neck can be influenced.

The position of the head at the moment of collision influences the type of injury. This is particularly true of the degree of rotation in relationship to the direction of impact. As shown in Figure 63, when the head faces directly forward, the uppermost vertebra glides forward on the one below and causes symmetrical narrowing of the spinal canal and symmetrical overriding of the facets. The intervertebral foramina are therefore closed equally in this maneuver. As Figure 74

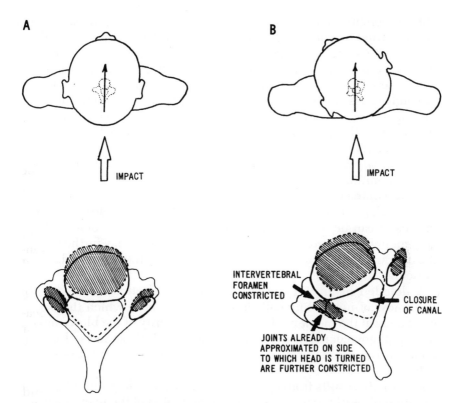

FIGURE 63. Effect of deceleration injury to neck with head turned. *A*, The "to-and-fro" movement of flexion and extension of a deceleration injury with the head facing forward. *B*, With the head rotated to left, the forward glide causes constriction of the foramen on the side toward which the head is turned. The foramen is already smaller (physiologically) on that side, and the joints are already in closer proximity. The spinal canal also undergoes greater deformity; thus more strain upon the spinal cord may result.

in Chapter 6 shows, the foramen are open equally when the head faces forward but are narrowed on the side toward which the head is laterally flexed or to which the head is turned. An oblique line of impact will combine flexion and extension with rotation and lateral flexion. Not only will the already narrowed foramen be compressed more, but the torque effect on the facets, capsules, and ligaments will be far more damaging. The effect on the intervertebral foramina and the spinal canal is demonstrated in Figure 63.

Pure dislocation is common in the cervical spine because very little flexion is necessary to disengage the articular processes. Pure flexion alone, however, rarely ruptures the posterior ligament complex. To tear these posterior structures, rotation is necessary.[8] In extension, the anterior longitudinal ligament tears to allow posterior dislocation; this is intensified by some degree of rotation. Unilateral facet dislocation occurs with vertebral body displacement through a distance of only half the anterior-posterior depth of the body. Forward displacement of one vertebral body of more than half[10] the anterior-posterior width of the body causes dislocation[11] of *both* facets and tearing of the annulus, the longitudinal ligaments, and the ligaments of the facets. Rotating the head at the time of collision increases the possibility of more serious injury.

Momentary awareness of the impending accident can protect the neck by minimizing the pendular action of the head on the neck. Muscle contraction spares the action imposed on the ligaments. If there is a lapse between the impact and the reflex muscle contraction, the result can be a compressive force applied at the moment of disalignment of the vertebrae. This compressive force may further distort the disk and the articular facets as well as irritate the periosteal sites of muscular attachment.

A detailed history of the accident as to direction of impact, the awareness of impending collision, the direction in which the person was facing at the moment of accident, the severity of the blow, and the resultant movements of the head and neck—all these facts obviously relate to the mechanism of injury and particularize the tissues envolved.

Local pain results from cervical sprain in a deceleration injury, and irritation of contiguous tissues within the region of the neck can cause *referred pain*. Irritation of cervical nerve roots through their foraminal passage evokes the specific clinical manifestations shown previously in Figures 49, 50 and 51. The way nerve roots can be affected has already been discussed. Suffice it to say here that any of the tissues forming and lining the intervertebral foramen are capable of compressing its contents. Intraspinal, intraforaminal, and extraspinal tissues all contribute to the picture.

The subluxation effect and the results of sprain have thus far been limited to the vertebrae between C_3 and C_7. Similar displacement can occur from fracture and dislocation between the atlas (C_1) and the axis (C_2) as shown in Figure 64. At this level there is potential injury to the spinal cord, the upper cervical nerves (Figs. 37, 65 and 66), and the vertebral arteries. Figure 64 also shows the many sites of possible fracture in lower cervical vertebrae and the tissues most commonly injured by these fractures.

Of all the symptoms resulting from cervical sprain injuries, the most confusing are those attributable to the sympathetic nervous system. The complex neuroanatomy of the sympathetic nervous system was presented in Figure 35. Involvement of the sympathetics may occur

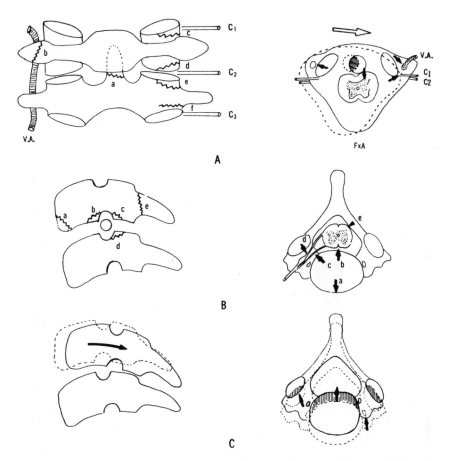

FIGURE 64. Sites of fracture-dislocations in the cervical spine. A, Fracture-dislocation sites: a, odontoid process; b, process; c–f, articular facets of atlas-axis. B, Fracture sites: letters show corresponding site in both views. C, Posterior dislocation sites (bilateral).

by stimulation of the posterior cervical sympathetics, by stimulation of the sensory elements of C_1 and C_2, by simultaneous sympathetic irritation during nerve root compression in its foraminal passage, by compression of the vertebral artery, or by encroachment of the basilar veins. Irritation may thus be intraforaminal or extravertebral.

The sympathetic symptoms are most frequently *aural*, such as tinnitus–occasionally with deafness–and postural dizziness, or *ocular*, with blurred vision, pain behind the eyeballs, and a dilated pupil on the involved side that dilates when the head is turned and returns to normal with the head in a neutral position. Other sympathetic symptoms claimed include corneal hypasthesia, miosis, rhinorrhea,

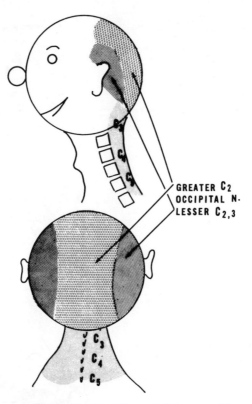

FIGURE 65. Dermatomal distribution of the occipital nerves. The greater occipital and lesser occipital nerves formed from roots C_2, C_3, and C_4 refer pain to the occipital vertex or parietal areas of the head as depicted by shaded areas.

sweating, lacrimation, and photophobia. The C_5 root contains fibers that join the carotid plexus; sympathetic fibers that accompany the C_6 root proceed to the subclavian artery and the brachial plexus; and the fibers along C_7 go to the cardiac, aortic, and phrenic plexi. The sympathetic nervous system plays a part in brachialgic (nerve-root-referred) pain, as evidenced from the relief that frequently follows cervical sympathetic blocks, periarterial sympathectomy, stellate ganglionectomy, and scalenotomy. Unfortunately for scientific verification, most symptoms of a sympathetic nature are subjective.

Patients sustaining a deceleration or acceleration accident may also undergo symptoms of cerebral concussion with momentary lapse of consciousness. At the time of collision they may feel a "blinding" or "explosive" sensation in the head. This may be followed immediately or several hours later by headache, restlessness, insomnia, mood changes, and signs of vasomotor instability. Again, these signs and

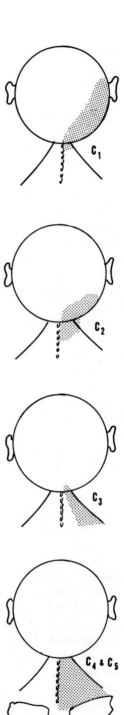

FIGURE 66. Referred zones of root levels. Injection of an irritant into paraspinous areas of the cervical spine (C_1 through C_5) results in pain noted by patients in the shaded areas.

89

symptoms are subjective and difficult to differentiate from psychoneurosis or malingering. The postconcussion syndrome remains an enigma.

SYNDROME OF ACUTE CENTRAL SPINAL CORD INJURY

The syndrome of the acute central spinal cord injury[12] is a severe neurological syndrome that may occur after a deceleration hyperflexion or hyperextension injury.

Patients have been known to sustain a severe neurological deficit after a hyperextension injury to the cervical spine with minimal or even no evidence of alteration of vertebral alignment. This pattern, characteristic of acute central cervical spinal cord injury, was originally attributed to cord contusion, as either a transient vertebral subluxation or a "squeezing" of the cord during hyperextension between the hypertrophic spur anteriorly and the posterior wrinkled ligamentum flavum (Fig. 67). The partial ("relative") transient insufficiency of the vertebral artery is now considered as another possible cause.

The "syndrome" reveals more motor impairment of the upper than of the lower extremities, possibly bladder dysfunction, and sensory loss below the level of the lesion. When the cord damage results in hemorrhage (hematomyelia) the symptoms may progress cephalad or caudad and may even result in death. When the damage is edema, gradual return of function usually occurs in a sequence: first, return of motor power in the lower extremities, then return of bladder function, and last, return of upper extremity strength to the very last finger. The initial sensory deficit does not follow any specific pattern but may vary from immediate, complete to all sensations, to *no* loss at all.

Whether the injury is cord "contusion" from compression or from "relative vascular insufficiency" is not always clear. In the former there is usually marked sensory as well as motor loss. The examination reveals posterior column and lateral spinothalamic damage with some sensory loss. The latter—i.e., the vascular impairment—has little or no long tract sensory impairment.

This syndrome is frequent in the elderly patient with degenerative osteoarthritis who sustains a "deceleration hyperextension cervical spine injury." The history may be the only conclusive evidence, with the symptoms absent at the time of examination.

In vertebral artery compression, the sites[13] are (1) fracture-dislocation above C_6, (2) atlanto-axial dislocation, or (3) the occipito-atlanto junction where the occipital condyle slides over C_1.

The typical case history is this: rear-end collision with the patient not striking his head nor losing consciousness; full awareness of the impact from behind; usually a sudden "snapping" back of the head

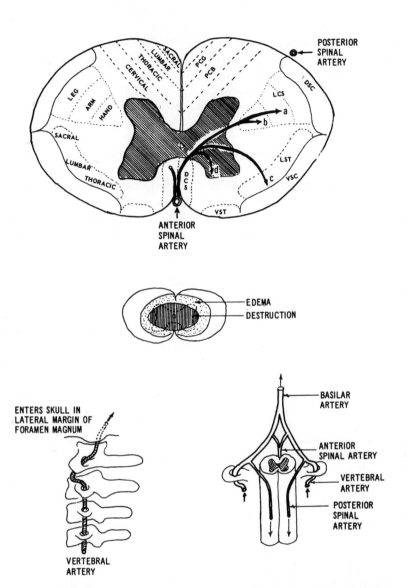

FIGURE 67. Vascular supply to the cervical cord. The arterial circulation that sustains a transient impairment in the syndrome of acute central spinal cord injury is shown. The clinical neurological symptoms are explained by the cord tracts that sustain the ischemia. *a* and *b*, Supply arm and hand area of lateral corticospinal (pyramidal) tract. *c*, Supplies lumbar and thoracic area of lateral spinothalamic tract. *d*, Supplies anterior medial portion of gray matter.

PCG = Posterior column Goll
PCB = Posterior column Burdach
DCS = Dorsal spinocerebellar
LCS = Lateral corticospinal

LST = Lateral spinothalamic
VSC = Ventral spinocerebellar
VST = Ventral spinothalamic
DSC = Direct corticospinal

and some neck symptoms. Immediately the patient feels "numbness" of the entire trunk and extremities and is unable to move either arms or legs; possibly some "tingling" of both arms or legs; inability to void; (objectively, on examination the sense of vibration, position, and light touch is preserved); return of power and sensation occurs as previously described.

DIAGNOSIS OF DECELERATION SPRAIN INJURY

Diagnosis demands a carefully detailed history and a thorough musculo-skeletal-neurological examination. Range of neck motion in the passive and the active range must be evaluated by comparison with what is normal. The symmetry, sequence, and site of neck movement as well as the extent must be analyzed. Whenever possible, the symptoms claimed must be verified by a careful neurological examination. The cranial nerves including ophthalmoscopic examination, deep reflexes, sensory dermatome mapping with comparison of one side with the other, motor strength—all these aspects of the examination will associate the subjective with objective findings. The history and symptoms claimed may be verified by examination.

X-rays must be carefully interpreted so that too much is not interpreted or misinterpreted. Abnormal findings may be unrelated to symptoms or clinical findings, just as definite signs and symptoms may exist in the presence of "negative" X-rays. The presence of "degenerative disk disease" on X-ray does not attribute all symptoms of the neck and upper extremities to "arthritis." Arthritic changes are long in coming and frequently have been completely asymptomatic. They indicate previous damage and attempts at repair. At best they may indicate a "point of weakness," but here, too, it is interesting that irritation of a nerve root can occur one level higher than the narrowed space which has an obviously restricted motion.

Following acute injury to the neck, X-rays are frequently read as revealing "straightening of the cervical lordosis." This position is thought to relieve pain (antalgic position), and it is attributed to muscle spasm or to wedging of protruded disk material in the posterior portion of the cervical spine so as to reverse the physiological lordosis. The exact mechanism is vague and the interpretation equivocal. Recent studies[14] claim this "straight cervical spine" to be due to positioning while taking the film, which claim is substantiated by finding a *straight spine to be normally curved* upon repeating X-rays *shortly* after the *initial* films with no intervening treatment or medication.

A reversed segmental curve in the neck X-rays is always more significant, since it may well indicate subluxation, ligamentous tear, acute disk herniation, or fracture. A full discussion of X-ray techniques and interpretation is beyond our scope here, but the point is that X-rays play an ancillary part in diagnosis—a valuable but a subsidiary role. Views should always include A-P, lateral, both obliques, and open-mouth views. Further views are demanded by the condition.

REFERENCES

1. The Revolt Against 'Whiplash'. The Defense Research Institute, P.O. Box 126, Union Station, Syracuse, New York.
2. Schutt, C. H. and Dohan, E. C.: Neck injuries to women in auto accidents. J.A.M.A. 206:2689–92, 1968.
3. Stedman's Medical Dictionary. Baltimore, Williams & Wilkins, 1976.
4. Fielding, J. W.: Cineroentgenography of the normal cervical spine. J. Bone Joint Surg. 39-A:1280–1, 1957.
5. Sherrington, C.: The Integrated Action of the Nervous System. Yale, 1947.
6. Basmajian, J. V. and Latif, A.: Integrated actions and functions of the chief flexors of the elbow: A detailed electromyographic analysis. J. Bone Joint Surg. 39A:1106–18, 1957.
7. Bard, P.: Medical Physiology. St. Louis, C. V. Mosby, 1956, p. 1028.
8. Roaf, R.: A study of the mechanics of spinal injuries. J. Bone Joint Surg. 42-B:810–23, 1960.
9. Cameron, B. M.: A 'Whiplash' symposium: Theory critique. Orthopedics 2:127–29, 1960.
10. Beatson, T. R.: Fracture and dislocations of the cervical spine. J. Bone Joint Surg. 45-B:21–35, 1963.
11. Holdsworth, F. W.: Fractures, dislocation and fracture dislocations of the spine. J. Bone Joint Surg. 45-B:6–20, 1963.
12. Schneider, R. C. and Schemm, G. W.: Vertebral artery insufficiency in acute and chronic spinal trauma, with special reference to the syndrome of acute central cervical spinal cord injury. J. Neurosurg. 18:348–60, 1961.
13. Schneider, R. C. and Crosby, E.C.: Vascular insufficiency of brain stem and spinal cord in spinal trauma. Neurology 9:643–56, 1960.
14. Juhl, J. H., Miller, S. M., and Roberts, G. W.: Roentgenographic variations in the normal cervical spine. Radiology, 78:591–7, 1962.

BIBLIOGRAPHY

Breig, A.: Biomechanics of the Central Nervous System. Chicago, Year Book Publishers, 1960.
Chrisman, O. D. and Gervais, R. F.: Otologic manifestations of the cervical syndrome. Clin. Orthop. 24:34–9, 1962.
McKeever, D. C.: The so-called whiplash injury. Orthopedics 2:14, 1960.
Stewart, D. Y.: Current concepts of the 'Barre syndrome' or the 'posterior cervical sympathetic syndrome.' Clin. Orthop. 24:40–8, 1962.

CHAPTER 6

Degenerative Disk Disease

Disk degeneration undoubtedly plays a greater role in the production of neck pain, nerve root pathology, or spinal cord compression than does acute disk herniation. Disk degeneration eventually occurs in man. It may be the end result of nuclear herniation, annular protrusion, or dehydration and fissure of the disk material and fibrous replacement of a degenerated annulus. Aging, stresses of daily living, movements and positions, injuries, and emotional tensions all have a detrimental effect upon the structure and nutrition of the disk. *Ultimately all disks undergo degenerative changes* of varying degrees.

The vascular supply of the normal disk is obliterated in the second decade of life, and nutrition from then on is by imbibition and osmosis. Which factors participate in the degenerative changes of the disk remain unknown. Someday research may prove that *normal* stresses imparted upon an *abnormal* disk cause the so-called degeneration and that the *abnormal* disk results from hereditary mutations,[1] childhood infections, metabolic enzyme alterations,[2] and so forth. Aging alone cannot explain disk degeneration, since cases of clinical herniation in the first decade of life[3] have been reported.

A satisfactory explanation of disk nutrition is that the nutritive fluids are imbibed by "spongelike" action of the disk contracting and expanding due to alterations of gravity and muscular action. The fluids thus brought to the disk are further imbibed by colloidal chemical action. This reasoning would explain partially the disk degeneration observed in people who are chronically emotionally tense, under persistent occupational tension, posturally tense, or whose general physical inflexibility decreases their circulatory integrity. This interesting concept gives reason to advocating exercise and periodic antigravity rest as well as traction to enhance nutrition and repair of the disk.

Degeneration of the disk is considered to begin within the annulus as slight tears in the annular fibers. This is followed or occurs simultaneously with softening of the nucleus. The nucleus, originally a firm yet elastic gel, undergoes fragmentation.

Initially the nuclear material remains encapsulated within the annular container but gradually forces its way peripherally through the tears of the annulus (Fig. 68). Protrusion continues, forcing the annulus to "bulge" peripherally which ultimately presses against the longitudinal ligaments causing them to separate from their attachments to the vertebral bodies (Fig. 69).

As the disk degenerates it also dehydrates and the intradiskal pressure decreases. This intradiskal pressure exerted caudally and cranially against the opposing vertebral end plates thus causing them to remain separated by its decreased nuclear pressure allows the vertebrae to approximate. This approximation occurs as the result of gravity and muscular tension.

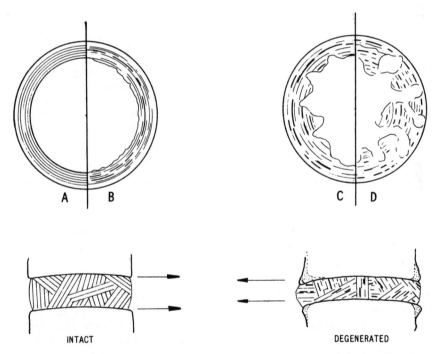

FIGURE 68. Evolutionary stages of disk degeneration. A, Young, intact disk with elastic annular fibers and a well hydrated nucleus. B, Early stages of degeneration reveal fibrillation of the annulus, some fragmentation, and beginning dehydration of the annulus. C, Moderate stage shows a furtherance of B with early invasion of the annulus by fragments of the nucleus. D, Advanced stage of degeneration is that of marked nuclear dehydration and fragmentation with invasion of the shredded annulus permitting nuclear fragments to reach the periphery of the disk where only the ligamentous structures remain.

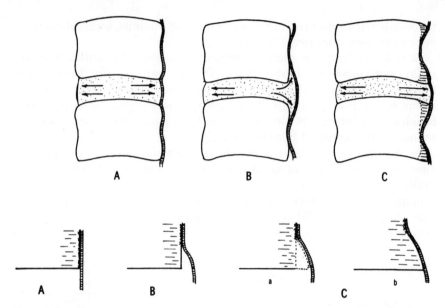

FIGURE 69. Mechanism of spondylosis. A, Normal anterior portion of functional unit with an intact disk, normal interspace, and a taut posterior longitudinal ligament that is totally adherent to the vertebral body periosteum. B, Disk degeneration permits approximation of the two vertebrae, causing a slack in the posterior longitudinal ligament. The intradiskal pressure dissects the ligament away from the periosteum, and disk material intervenes. C, Extruded disk material becomes fibrous, a, then calcifies into a "spur," b.

There is sufficient residual intradiskal pressure within the nucleus to exert pressure peripherally to force annular and disk matrix tissue against the longitudinal ligaments to further dissect the ligaments away from the vertebral bodies. This disk material, annular and matrix, is forced into the space between the body and the dissected ligament—veritably a "bulge."

This protruding disk material is often called a "soft" disk herniation. Ultimately there is a preponderance of annular material with increasing fibrous tissue invasion firming the protusion. This is now termed a "hard" disk herniation. If there is further repair, as there usually is, the bulge undergoes calcification and forms a calcific spur or an "osteophyte" (see Fig. 69).

Approachment of the vertebral bodies also approximates the posterolateral protrusions called the *uncovertebral joints of von Luschka.* The true anatomy and physiology of these "joints" is controversial.[4] Synovial lining, synovial fluid, and a joint capsule existing in these joints is denied by most anatomists. Rather, they are considered to be bony protrusions arising along the posterior lateral border of the ver-

96

tebral bodies that, over the years, through friction and abrasion become smooth surfaces. As they have no articular surfaces, no joint capsules, and no synovial fluid, they are essentially *pseudoarthroses*.

In their function as joints with constant irritation and friction they also become the site of osteophyte formation (Fig. 70). These hypertrophic changes of "spondylosis" ultimately affect the entire periphery of the involved vertebrae. The central bulging from osteophytosis under the longitudinal ligament and the thickening of the uncovertebral joints may form an osteophytic bridge or spur completely across the rim of the vertebra and encroach into the spinal canal (Fig. 71).

Approximation of the anterior portion of the functional unit inevitably reapproaches the posterior articulations, and by approachment there is loss of congruity of the joint surfaces and compression of the cartilaginous articular surfaces. The normal nutrition and lubrication

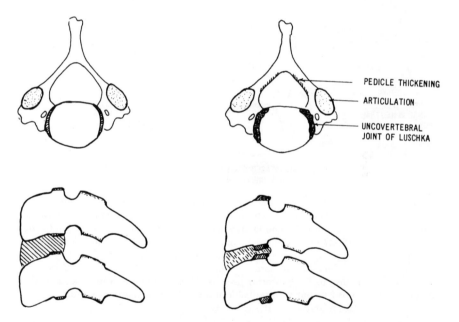

PEDICLE THICKENING

ARTICULATION

UNCOVERTEBRAL
JOINT OF LUSCHKA

FIGURE 70. Disk degeneration with formation of "spondylosis." *Left,* Normal relationship of the vertebral bodies separated by an intact disk, normal uncovertebral joints of von Luschka, and normal posterior articulations (facets). *Right,* Changes resulting from disk degeneration. The vertebral bodies approximate; the uncovertebral joints thicken, roughen, and distort; the foramina deform; and the facets thicken and also deform. These drawings do not show the additional soft tissue changes such as thickening of the longitudinal ligaments and thickening and curling of the ligamentum flavum. The facet capsules also thicken. All these soft tissue changes plus the bony changes shown narrow the intervertebral foramina and the interspinal canal.

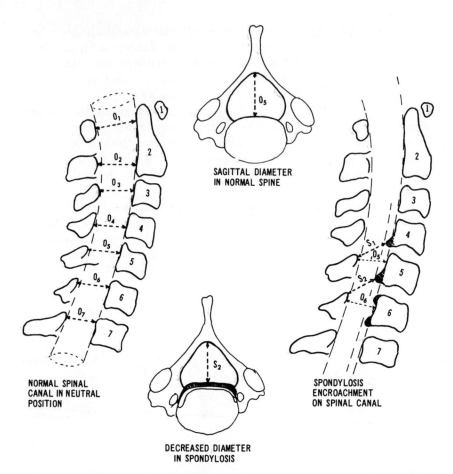

NORMAL SPINAL
CANAL IN NEUTRAL
POSITION

SAGITTAL DIAMETER
IN NORMAL SPINE

DECREASED DIAMETER
IN SPONDYLOSIS

SPONDYLOSIS
ENCROACHMENT
ON SPINAL CANAL

FIGURE 71. Sagittal diameter of the cervical spinal canal. From X-rays, the lateral view depicts the sagittal (anterior-posterior) diameter of the cervical bony canal. In the neutral position of the normal spine O_1 averages 22 mm; O_2, 20 mm; and C_3 to C_7 are constant between 12–22 mm (average 17 mm). Neck extension from full flexion may alter the diameter by 2 mm. Spondylosis narrows the canal diameter (S_1 and S_2). This measurement is from the posterior border of one vertebra to the upper border of the next lower laminal junction to the posterior process. Cord compression may occur if the diameter is 10 mm or less but is improbable if it is 13 mm or more. See text.

of these zygapophyseal joints are shown in Figure 72. The mechanism of deformity through osteoarthritic changes is depicted in Figure 73.

Degenerative changes in the cervical spine evolving from the disk changes deform the intervertebral foramina as well as the size and shape of the spinal canal. Normal variations in the size of the intervertebral foraminal openings are depicted in Figure 74. Degenerative

98

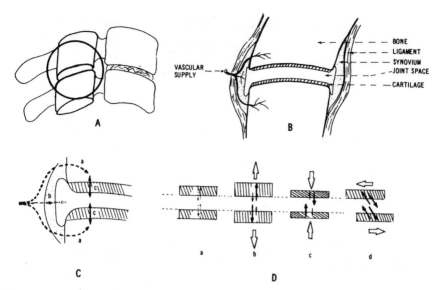

FIGURE 72. Normal nutrition and lubrication of posterior articulation (facet). A, The posterior articulation, the zygapophyseal joint. This cervical joint is a diarthroidial joint containing a capsule, synovium, joint space containing fluid, and two articular cartilages; it is supplied by its unique vascular bed, B. C, Diffusion cycle to cartilage nutrition. The arterial supply separates into a capillary bed to bone, a, and a capillary bed to the synovium, b. Cartilage nutrition is by diffusion through the cartilage, c, from both capillary beds by "spongelike" compression and expansion of the cartilage. D, Mechanism of cartilage nutrition. a, No imbibition with joint at rest. b, Inflow from relaxation or joint extension. c, "Squeezing" out of synovial fluid by cartilage compression. d, Creation of lubrication layer between surfaces by motion between two incongruent surfaces.

changes make these variations greater and potentially compressive to the tissues in the foramina.

The predominant sites of osteophyte formation in the entire spine are at the summits of concavity,[5] at the points farthest from the center of gravity. As shown in Figure 75, these sites are at C_4–C_5 and C_5–C_6 in the cervical region, at T_8 in the thoracic spine, and at L_3–L_4 in the lumbar lordosis. These findings lead to the concept that osteophytes develop as a defense mechanism and thus are a *repair* process rather than a disease state. The osteophytes ultimately are composed of more compact strong bone than is the rest of the vertebral body. Their intended *repair* function is marred by their potential damage from protrusion into the spinal canal and the intervertebral foramina.

The most disk degeneration appears in the lordotic curves which form as a result of man's erect posture. These curves have the greatest *static* stress; since these areas (lordosis) also have the greatest move-

99

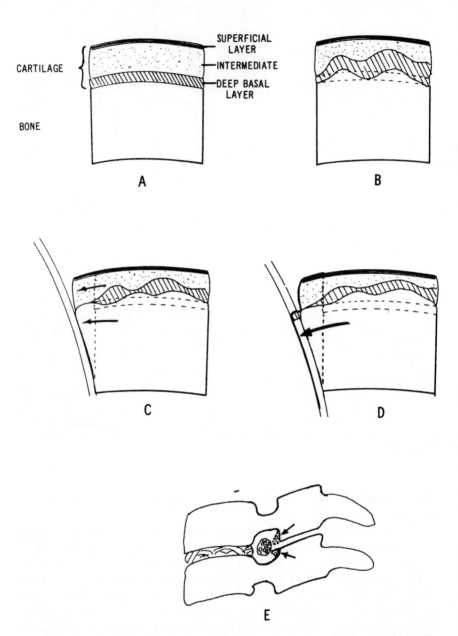

FIGURE 73. Mechanism of osteoarthritic changes in facet joints. A, The articular cartilage consists of three layers: (1) superficial tangential layer of collagen fibers, (2) an
intermediate spongy, shock-absorbing layer, and (3) a deep, calcified, basal layer that is
firmly bound to the subchondral bone. B, Wear and tear causes new bone formation of
the subchondral plate and thickening of the calcified basal layer with lengthening of the
bone. C, Peripheral lateral growth widens the end of the bone, and finally, D, the
ligaments ossify. E, Encroachment into the intervertebral foramen from osteoarthritis.

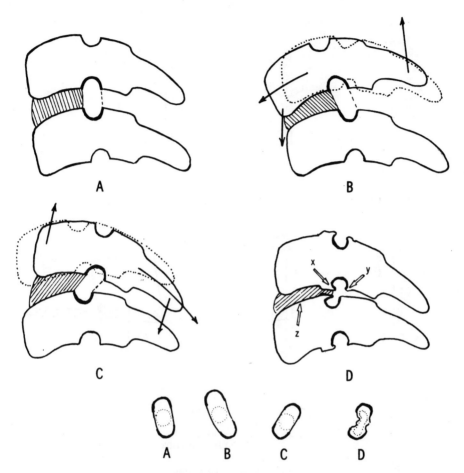

FIGURE 74. Foraminal opening variations. A, Normal open intervertebral foramen with the neck in a neutral, slightly flexed position and not rotated or laterally tilted to either side. B, Flexion, which occurs below C_3 by forward gliding of the upper upon the lower vertebra, maintains full opening. C, Extension by backward gliding of the upper upon the lower vertebra normally narrows the foraminal aperture. D, Degenerated disk and osteophyte formation from the joints of von Luschka (not even considering the soft tissue components). Comparison with normal, A, shows the marked encroachment upon the foraminal space.

ment, they are the sites of maximum *kinetic* stress as well. Trauma in this respect undoubtedly plays a part in disk degeneration and in its repair mechanism.

Anterior osteophytes occur most often in the thoracic spine, whereas the *posterior* osteophytes prevail in the cervical (and lumbar) spine. This conforms to the concept of greatest pressure on the con-

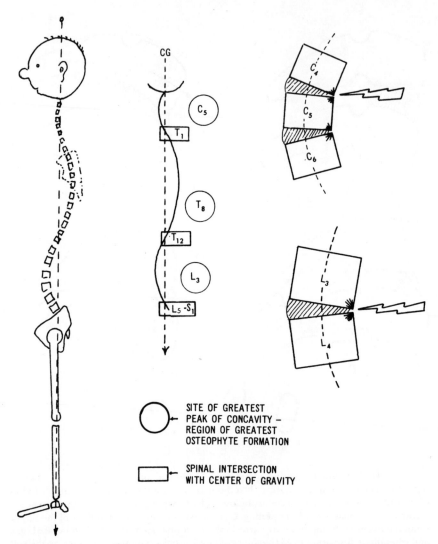

FIGURE 75. Sites of greatest osteophyte formation. The lateral view of the static erect spine (posture) demonstrates the sites of transection of the spine with the plumb line of gravity (external ear meatus, odontoid process, T_1, T_{12}, and sacral promontory). The greatest points of pressure, thus the sites of osteophyte formation, are at the points of greatest concavity, farthest from the plumb line (C_5, T_8, L_3).

cave side of the curve and to the freer extension movement of the cervical spine.

Faulty posture can accelerate degenerative changes. Poor posture in which the dorsal kyphosis is accentuated and the compensatory superincumbent cervical curve thus increased (extended) brings in all the factors that influence osteophyte formation (Figs. 76 and 77).

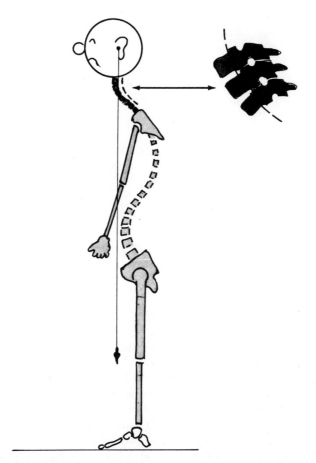

FIGURE 76. Effect of posture upon the cervical spine. The slumped forward posture causes the head to be held ahead of the center of gravity. The cervical spine must assume a greater lordosis to balance and thus closes the intervertebral foramina and places more pressure upon the zygoapophyseal (facet) joints.

Trauma upon a *normal* spine is adequately handled by elastic disks, resilient ligaments, elastic capsule tissue, and openings for nerve and blood vessels that have a good margin of safety. Trauma to a degenerated spine finds less compressibility in the disk, less reversible distortion of the disk, ligaments much less resilient, and foramen already narrowed to the point of a smaller margin of safety. The pre-existence of degeneration may have been quiescent in that no symptoms were noted, but now minor trauma may "decompensate" the safety margin and symptoms occur.

Degenerative changes occur in asymptomatic people as well as in patients with symptoms. The relationship of symptoms to radiological evidence of degeneration has not been, and is not always, established.

103

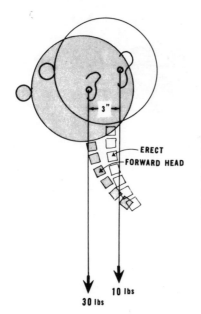

ERECT
FORWARD HEAD

10 lbs
30 lbs

FIGURE 77. Gravity effect upon the cervical spine. With erect posture, the weight of the head (approximately 10 pounds) is held directly above the center of gravity. In a forward head posture, the head is held inches ahead of the center of gravity and weighs the weight of the head *times* the inches ahead of the center, viz: 3″ = 30 lb, 4″ = 40 lb.

The presence of osteophytes invading the intervertebral foramina does not necessarily cause nerve root irritation as claimed by some,[6] nor does their absence exclude nerve root irritation.[7] In asymptomatic patients, 25 percent in their fifth decade show degenerative changes radiologically; by the seventh decade, 75 percent show changes.[8] Degeneration of the zygapophyseal joints can occur *without* significant disk degeneration, which indicates that this form of degeneration occurs due to alteration of the mechanics of the cervical spine.[9, 10] When zygapophyseal joint arthritis occurs in relationship to disk deneration it usually follows the disk desease by 10 years. Degenerative changes are slow which undoubtedly permits the nerves to adjust to entrapment and deformation without symptoms. Trauma intervenes in the form of mechanical injury, physical stress, or emotional strain, and the adaptation is overwhelmed, the defense is overcome and symptoms result. A good compensatory equilibrium requires a moderate to large stress to be overcome; if the equilibrium is tenuous, a minor stress will have great repercussions.

The site and the extent of degenerative disk disease with its secondary manifestations, either reparative or overwhelmed, will determine the site of the symptoms, imply the mechanism which is causing the symptoms, and relate the physical findings to the pathology. The symptoms may be pain felt locally and associated with limitation of neck movement, which would localize the pathological changes in the tissues of the posterior portion of the functional unit, primarily the apophyseal joint capsules, the ligaments, and the muscles. Symptoms related to neck movements but referred distally into the upper back, shoulders, and upper extremities implicate the intervertebral foramen and all its contiguous tissues. Signs and symptoms attributed to neck origin but referred distally as spinal cord involvement point to narrowing of the spinal canal in the neck region and encroachment of its contents.

The localizing characteristics associated with causation of symptoms imply *inadequate space* or *irritation from movement*. The history and physical examination will indicate the pain-producing posture, position, or movement. The examination will indicate a localization of the pain site. Properly interpreted tests will substantiate the anatomico-pathological condition suspected. The diagnosis will be established and proper treatment indicated.

REFERENCES

1. Clarke, E. and Little, J. H.: Cervical myelopathy: A contribution to its pathogenesis. Neurology 5:861–7, 1955.
2. Odom, G. L., Finney, W., and Woodhall, B.: Cervical disk lesions. J.A.M.A. 166:23–8, 1958.
3. King, A. B.: Surgical removal of a ruptured intervertebral disc in early childhood. J. Pediat. 55:57–62, 1959.
4. Orofino, C., Sherman, M. S., and Schechter, D.: Luschka's joint—A degenerative phenomenon. J. Bone Joint Surg. 42-A:853–8, 1960.
5. Nathan, H.: Osteophytes of the vertebral column. J. Bone Joint Surg. 44-A:243–68, 1962.
6. Friedenberg, Z. B. and Miller, W. T.: Degenerative disc disease of the cervical spine. J. Bone Joint Surg. 45-A:1171–8, 1963.
7. Tapiovaara, J. and Heinivaara, A.: Correlation of cervico-brachialgia and roentgenographic findings. Ann. Chir. Gynecol. Fenn. Suppl. 43:436–44, 1954.
8. Brain, W. R., Knight, G. C., and Bull, J. W. D.: Discussion of the intervertebral disk in the cervical region. Proc. R. Soc. Med. 41:509–16, 1948.
9. Horwitz, T.: Degenerative lesions in the cervical portion of the spine. Arch. Int. Med. 65:1178, 1940.
10. Holt, S. and Yates, P. O.: Cervical spondylosis and nerve root lesions. J. Bone Joint Surg. 48-B:407–23, 1966.

CHAPTER 7

Cervical Spondylotic Myelopathy

Cervical disk disease is accepted as a frequent cause of root symptoms. Frequently cervical diskogenic disease causes spinal cord impairment as well as root signs. The ensuing neurological deficit is of upper motor neuron involvement.

Cervical spondylotic myelopathy (CSM) was initially clarified from myelopathy due to acute disk prolapse in 1956.[1] Cervical spondylotic myelopathy is considered to be the most common neurological spinal cord disorder after middle age.[2] It must be remembered, however, that many patients with marked cervical spondylosis never develop symptoms and many who develop symptoms of myelopathy have little radiological evidence of spondylosis.

The principal pathology is encroachment of pathological tissue into the spinal canal or the intervertebral foramen or foraminae, or both. The exact mechanism of the cord involvement is not fully understood but there are sufficiently studied and accepted concepts to permit accurate diagnosis and meaningful therapy. The most acceptable theory of etiology is that critically large chondro-osseous spurs and movement equals progressive signs and symptoms of CSM.[3] Motion appears to be causative. The material that encroaches into the canal and/or foramen may be disk material or proliferating degenerated tissue (see Chapter 6). Soft central disk herniation, as opposed to cervical spondylosis, is an uncommon cause of myelopathy. Soft disks comprise only 1 to 2 percent of all operations performed for disks or bars.[4]

The normal spinal canal, in the midcervical region, is oval with an average sagittal diameter of 14 mm and 17 mm wide. The cervical cord at this level has a maximal sagittal diameter of 10 mm in the adult. The sagittal diameter of the canal increases with neck flexion and decreases with neck extension.[5] The canal, or the foramina, may be narrowed or angulated by a subluxation or dislocation. Change in the canal width may also be altered by movement or posture. These signs can be suspected and verified by a careful clinical examination, proper X-ray studies or myelography. If the protrusion or occlusion is in the direction of the foramen, root signs are manifested. If the protrusion is into the spinal canal, cord signs (upper motor neuron) are manifested (see Fig. 44). Myelopathy without root signs is relatively uncommon. Pain radiating down the arms and demonstrating hypalgesia, hypathesia or anesthesia of a dermatome distribution indicate involvement of a nerve root in the foramen.

Pain Terms: A list with definitions and notes on usage. Recommended by the IASP Subcommittee on Taxonomy (Pain 6:249–252, 1979).

Pain	An unpleasant sensory and emotional experience associated with actual or potential tissue damage, or described in terms of such damage.
Analgesia	Absence of pain or noxious stimulation.
Hyperalgesia	Diminished sensitivity to noxious stimulation.
Hyperaesthesia	Increased sensitivity to stimulation excluding special senses.
Hypoalgesia	Diminished sensitivity to noxious stimulation.
Neuralgia	Pain in the distribution of a nerve or nerves.
Neuritis	Inflammation of a nerve or nerves.
Neuropathy	A disturbance of function or pathological change in a nerve: in one nerve, mononeuropathy; in several nerves, mononeuropathy multiplex; symmetrical and bilateral, polyneuropathy.
Pain tolerance level	The greatest stimulus intensity causing pain that a subject is prepared to tolerate.

Damage to the cord will produce symptoms or findings dependent upon the specific tract or tracts involved (Fig. 78). Myelopathy has been attributed to direct pressure upon the cord or as a result of vascular impairment.[6-8]

The spinal cord receives its arterial supply from the anterior spinal artery and paired posterolateral arteries (Fig. 79). The anterior spinal artery receives blood from radicular arteries. Radicular arteries originate from vertebral and deep cervical vessels. They pass intradurally through the cervical neural foramina closely adjacent to the spinal nerve roots. The anterior spinal artery is usually a single vessel and is contained in the middle groove of the cord. This artery descends from "Y" bifurcation of the vertebral arteries[9] (Fig. 80; see also Fig. 67). The anterior spinal artery supplies the central gray area of the cord and the anterolateral white matter. Small branches go to the posterior cord to join branches of the paired posterior spinal arteries. The posterior spinal arteries zigzag and are not placed under traction in neck flexion. This apparently explains why the anterior columns and the outer half of the posterior columns are rarely affected.[10]

During laminectomy, the cord was seen to blanch from flexion of the neck.[11] Pathological changes in the cord were formed primarily in the area of the cord supplied by the anterior spinal artery.[7]

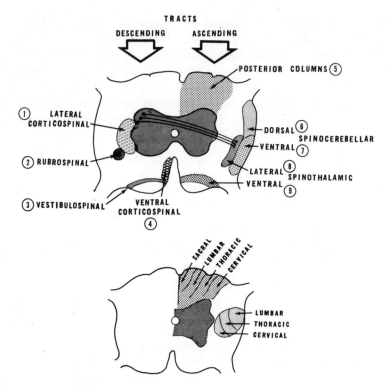

FIGURE 78. Sensory and motor tracts of the spinal cord. *Top*, generally, the descending tracts (1, 2, 3, and 4) are motor or for coordination and the ascending tracts (5, 6, 7, 8, and 9) carry sensation from the periphery to the higher centers. The ascending tracts convey the sensations of pain, touch, proprioception, and discrimination for interpretation. *Bottom*, areas of the extremities conveyed by the ascending (dotted area) and descending (lumbar, thoracic, and cervical) tracts.

Myelopathy has been attributed to direct pressure upon the cord from a sharp angulation of the canal causing traction or friction upon the cord. This defect may also be associated with narrowing of the width of the spinal canal (see Fig. 71). Rotation of the neck in the lower cervical region moves the zygapophyseal joints and the spurs within the foramina, compressing the dura, roots, and blood vessels within. This repeated trauma may lead to fibrosis. The veins may be occluded increasing the edema in the cord. The gross and microscopic pathological changes due to ischemia are greatest in the central gray and anterolateral white matter.[5]

A congenital narrowing of the sagittal diameter of the cervical spinal canal has been noted in patients who develop cervical spine myelopathy as compared with the general population.[12, 13] The exact measurement of the spinal canal diameter that has significance is not

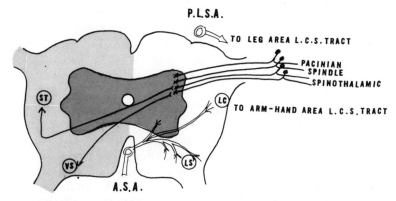

FIGURE 79. Spinal cord arterial supply. The posteriolateral spinal artery (PLSA) supplies the lateral corticospinal (LCS) tract to the leg area. The anterior spinal artery (ASA) supplies the region of the cord that contains the lateral corticospinal tract of the arm-hand area. The sensory roots entering the cord contain fibers from end organs within the extremities.

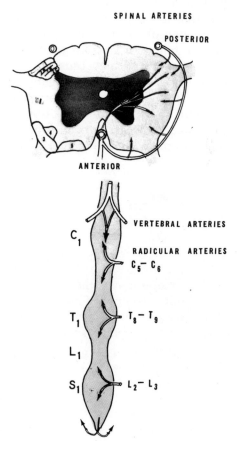

FIGURE 80. Spinal arterial supply. *Top,* the areas of the spinal cord that are supplied by the posterior and anterior spinal arteries are shown. Areas 1, 2A, 2B, and 2C are the sensory areas of the Lissauer tracts and the substantia gelatinosa. Areas 3, 4, and 5 are the spinothalamic, spinocerebellar, and coricospinal tracts. *Bottom,* the major radicular arterial branches of the spinal arteries are shown.

yet completely established[3] nor is the technique for X-ray studies standardized. The canal may be narrowed with compression of the cord during neck extension or hyperextension due to folding and bulging of the ligamentum flavum[14] (Fig. 81). The intrusion of the spines into the canal further narrows the canal diameter and must be considered in measurement.

Cervical spondylotic myelopathy has been reported to progress after successful surgical decompression. This has been attributed to excessive movement of the spine causing a tethering effect upon the nerves and the cord. Late deterioration, after successful surgery, may well occur from adhesions developing between the dural sac and the laminectomy scar. The cord is fixed cranially at the foramen magnum and caudally by the adhesions of the dural sac to the wall of the spinal canal. The dentate ligaments further fix the cord. The cord has markedly restricted movement, thus flexion of the neck, which elongates the canal, places traction upon the cord. Patients who have limited or no movement of the neck after surgical decompression are reported to not progress in their deterioration.[15, 16]

Any neurological tissue injury makes that tissue more susceptible to further injury. Excessive traction or compression upon an already traumatized cord may cause further myelopathy. The original cord damage (myelopathy) causing long tract signs may be followed by root signs. This additional symptomatology may be explained by repeated traction upon the roots by fibrosis of the nerve roots within the foramina, by vascular occlusion within the foramina, or by traction injury to the cord at the anterior and posterior gray horns[17] (Fig. 82).

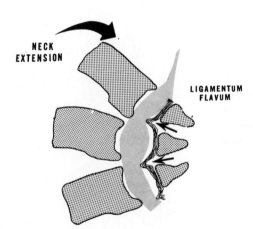

NECK
EXTENSION

LIGAMENTUM
FLAVUM

FIGURE 81. Spinal canal stenosis on neck extension. The spinal canal width may be further narrowed by neck extension due to the pleating of the ligamentum flavum.

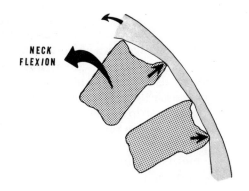

FIGURE 82. Spinal canal stenosis on neck flexion. In cervical spine forward flexion in the presence of spondylosis (osteophytic spurs) the cord and its dural sheath are subjected to traction and compression, thus decreasing the width of the canal.

NECK FLEXION

SYMPTOMS

Symptomatology may be insidious and extremely variable as to the neurological findings. The initial complaints may be of an unsteady gait or a feeling of "numbness" in the trunk and the extremities. "Weakness" may be complained of in the legs or the upper extremities.[18] Atrophy of the intrinsic muscles of the hand may be present but may indicate root entrapment from osteophyte invasion of the foramina as well as cord damage. Spasticity with or without weakness in the lower extremities is a frequent feature. Spasticity may be striking while weakness may be minimal.[19]

Pain is not usual. Rather a feeling of discomfort is claimed. Hypersensitivity of the hands or the feet may be the presenting symptoms. Urinary tract signs may be present, varying from dribbling to retention. Weakness, numbness, or hypersensitivity are not usually segmental or clearly delineated. A dermatomal pattern implicates a root rather than a myelopathy.[20] Impairment of pain and temperature may be volunteered by the patient or elicited on subsequent questioning. Objectively, this impairment may be striking. Dorsal column impairment is infrequent but can be identified by careful examination.[21] "Clumsiness" of finger movements is a frequent complaint and a certain percentage of patients with cervical myelopathy have impairment of the spinothalmic tracts (pain and temperature abnormality) with paresthesia.

Progression is usually not steady but appears to be a series of episodes from which new signs and symptoms appear but with *no complete remissions*. This latter fact helps differentiate it from multiple sclerosis.

111

PROGNOSIS

Advanced age with a short duration of symptoms before decompression has a poorer prognosis for recovery. Intrinsic hand muscle atrophy is also unfavorable, whereas severe lower extremity spasticity is not necessarily unfavorable. Sphincter loss is a poor prognostic sign as is significant lower extremity weakness. Loss of bladder and bowel control has been reversible following surgery.[16] Fine hand movement improves after surgery in many cases. Debate continues considering the merits of anterior surgical approach as compared with the posterior approach.

EXAMINATION

Long tract signs are predominant. Reflexes may be hyperactive and patient may have positive Babinski and Hoffman signs implicating pyramidal tract impairment. Gait may be spastic or ataxic. There may be hypalgesia below a specific cervical level. Position sense (MJT) may be impaired as well as vibration sense. Two point discrimination can be abnormal.

LABORATORY FINDINGS

Spinal fluid protein is frequently elevated. X-rays of the cervical spine may reveal encroachment upon the spinal canal or subluxation of one vertebral body upon the adjacent vertebra. In viewing spinal films, the sagittal diameter must be measured (see Fig. 71). This is measured from the middle of the posterior surface of the vertebra body to the nearest point of the junction of the lamina and the apex (Fig. 83). If there is subluxation (listhesis) viewed with X-rays taken in full flexion and full extension, this is measured in millimeters. This distance is measured from the posterior border of one vertebral body as compared with the posterior border of the adjacent vertebra (Fig. 84).

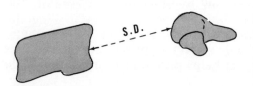

FIGURE 83. Spinal canal width. In measuring the anterior-posterior width of the spinal canal, the spinal diameter (SD) measures the distance between the posterior margin of the vertebral body and the anteriormost margin of the lamina and zygapophyseal joint.

FIGURE 84. Measurement of subluxation. The extent of subluxation (S) can be measured by comparing the hindmost protrusion of the vertebral body projecting into the spinal canal with the similar protrusion of an adjacent vertebral body.

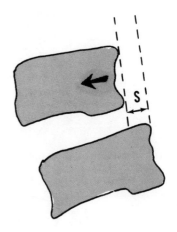

The spinal canal width averages 11.8 mm (9 to 15 mm) at the axis, where osteophytes do not occur the width averages 19.2 cm. Myelopathy occurs here in widths less than 17.2 mm.[22, 23] Although a congenitally narrow canal per se does not cause myelopathy it predisposes to it. When paraparesis does occur from protruding osteophytes, disk material, or subluxation, it is more severe in a patient with pre-existing congenital narrowing.[24]

The range of motion of the neck from extension to flexion is measured as the amount of kyphosis and lordosis in millimeters from the base of the skull to the seventh cervical vertebra[25] (Fig. 85). In evaluating flexion-extension films of the cervical spine, segmental movement or lack of segmented movement (e.g., C_4 upon C_5) must be noted and related to clinical signs. Subluxation of a vertebra may only be noted upon flexion-extension films.

MYELOGRAPHY

Pantopaque myelography has been largely replaced by water soluble dyes or by air myelography. Pantopaque, besides being incriminated in the production of arachnoiditis, is too heavy to fill interstices and, thus, does not give a complete picture.[26] Also, the position of hyperextension needed to prevent pantopaque from entering the intracranial cavity is not well tolerated by the patient and prolongs the examination. Carefully interpreted, a myelogram depicts the width of the canal, reveals encroachment of the canal by disk, osteophytes, bulging ligamentum flavum angulation from a subluxed vertebra, and so forth. These findings correlated with the clinical findings clarify the pathology and indicate the level of the lesion.

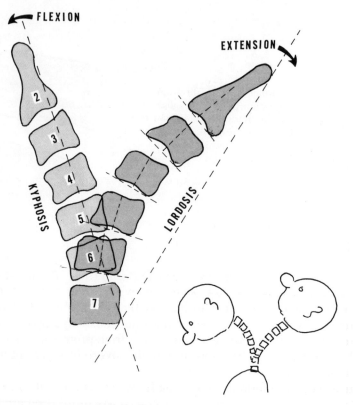

FIGURE 85. Measurement of cervical spine flexion-extension. Superimposition of flexion X-rays upon lateral extension views (superimposing C_7) may be used to compare segmental differences. Extension causes a central lordosis; flexion a kyphosis.

Degenerative changes are common in the cervical spines of people over age 50. It is assumed that this is "expected and of no significance." A significant diagnosis of *cervical spondylosis* must be made with certain physical signs, skeletal and neurological, as well as confirmed radiological abnormalities. Observation and treatment must be based on the presence or potential of symptoms and abnormal physical signs.[27]

The abnormal radiological findings are: canal narrowing due to (a) posterior osteophytes, (b) subluxation of one vertebra upon the adjacent vertebra, and (c) loss of the cervical lordosis at one segment (functional unit).

Clinically, there may be restricted neck movement mostly in lateral flexion and rotation. Reproduction of symptoms is not expected unless a Lhermitte's sign is elicted. Radicular pain on neck extension does

114

not confirm myelopathy. Neurological findings are frequently found that have not been clinically apparent or disabling. These include:

1. Abnormal reflexes in *upper* extremities (Hoffmann and exaggerated deep reflexes).
2. Exaggerated deep tendon reflexes in lower extremities.
3. Impaired vibration sensation in lower extremities (posterior column).

Impaired sensory loss in the upper extremities is difficult to differentiate from root signs secondary to foraminal narrowing. In the lower extremities, a coincidental lumbar spondylosis can confuse the picture of cervical spondylosis.

A positive Babinski sign has been reported in many asymptomatic people over age 50.[28, 29] None were attributed to cervical spondylosis but may have been. They should be followed carefully for early intervention when other signs of progression or disability appear. There may be *no* further narrowing of the canal so the neurological findings are important. Impaired vibration sense has also been found with increasing frequency in persons over age 50.[30] This has also not been correlated with cervical cord pathology. Arm reflexes such as a unilateral isolated absence of a deep tendon jerk (BJ or TJ) has been related to cord impairment but this is difficult to differentiate from lower motor neuron impairment at the foramina. EMG testing is available for this differentiation if its presence presents a diagnostic problem. A positive Hoffman sign indicates upper motor neuron disease (pyramidal tract) of the cord.

In essence, a patient over 50 with radiological findings of cervical canal narrowing, clinical findings of neck range of motion limitation, and neurological findings consistent with cord involvement has *symptomatic cervical spondylosis with myelopathy* and needs further diagnostic studies, careful observation and possibly therapeutic intervention.

TREATMENT

There are many reports crediting immobilization as effective.[1] This requires immobilization of the head and neck in the proper flexed angle to insure the appropriate elongation of the canal as well as the opening of the foramina. Movement must be eliminated or markedly restricted. All aspects of immobilization are discussed in Chapter 8. Periodic, careful, well documented examination must be assured to ascertain improvement or progression. Traction is of little value in treatment of myelopathy.

Indications for surgery are the presence of chronic, unremitting radicular pain, chronic cervical pain accompanied by radicular numbness, or progressive decline in spinal cord function.[3] Surgical decompression may be by posterior or anterior approach or anterior interbody fusion—all have their advocates and this issue will not be resolved in this text. It appears desirable that a surgical procedure not only decompress but also realign the canal and limit motion.[32] Immediately postoperatively and for a long period (three to six months) the neck must be immobilized in a firm support and no attempt at increasing range of motion must be considered. Improvement of posture, decrease of cervical lordosis, and avoidance of daily frequent hyperextension must be assured (see Chapter 8, Treatment).

REFERENCES

1. Taylor, A. R.: Vascular factors in the myelopathy associated with cervical spondylosis. Neurology 14:62, 1964.
2. Brain, W. R., Northfield, D., and Wilkinson, M.: Spondylosis: The known and the unknown. Lancet I:687, 1954.
3. Schneider, R. C., Cherry, B., and Pantek, H.: The syndrome of acute central cervical cord injury with special reference to the mechanics involved in hyperextension injuries of the cervical spine. J. Neurosurg. II:546–77, 1954.
4. Scoville, W. B.: Types of cervical disc lesions and their surgical approaches. J.A.M.A. 196:479–81, 1966.
5. Hoff, J., et al.: The role of ischemia in the pathogenesis of cervical spondylotic myelopathy. Spine 2:2, 1977.
6. Morton, D. E.: A comparative anatomico-roentgenological study of the cervical spines of twelve cadavers. Am. J. Roentgenol. 63:523, 1950.
7. Mair, W. G. P. and Druckman, R.: The pathology of spinal cord lesions and their relation to the clinical fractures on protrusion of cervical intervertebral discs (a report of four cases). Brain 76:70–91, 1953.
8. Breig, A. and Turnbull, H. O.: Effects of mechanical stresses on the spinal cord in cervical spondylosis: A study of fresh cadaver material. J. Neurosurg. 25:45, 1966.
9. Chakravorty, B. G.: Arterial supply of the cervical spinal cord and its relation to the cervical myelopathy in spondylosis. Ann. R. Coll. Surg. 45:232–51, 1969.
10. Robinson, R. A., et al.: Cervical spondylotic myelopathy: Etiology and treatment concept. Spine 2:89–99, 1977.
11. Allen, K. L.: Neuropathies caused by long spurs in the cervical spine with special reference to surgical treatment. J. Neurol. Neurosurg. Psychiat. 15:20–36, 1952.
12. Wilkinson, H. A., et al.: Roentgenographic correlations in cervical spondylosis. Am. J. Roentgenol. 105:370–74, 1969.
13. Bradley, W. G. and Banna, M.: The cervical dural canal. A study of the "tight dural canal" and of syrengomyelia by prone and supine myelography. Br. J. Radiol. 41:608–14, 1968.
14. Taylor, A. R.: Mechanism and treatment of spinal and disorders associated with cervical spondylosis. Lancet I:717–20, 1953.
15. Bradshaw, P.: Some aspects of cervical spondylosis. Quart. J. Med. 26:177–208, 1957.

16. Adams, C. B. T. and Lague, V.: Studies in cervical spondylotic myelopathy. III: Some functional effects of operations for cervical spondylotic myelopathy. Brain 94:587–94, 1971.
17. Reid, J. D.: Effects of flexion-extension movements of the head and spine upon the spinal cord and nerve roots. J. Neurol. Neurosurg. Psychiat. 23:214–21, 1960.
18. Brain, W. R., Northfield, D. W., and Wilkinson, M.: The neurological manifestations of cervical spondylosis. Brain 75:187–225, 1952.
19. Bucy, P. C., Heimberger, R. F., and Aberhill, H. R.: Compression of the cervical spinal cord by herniated intervertebral discs. J. Neurosurg. 5:471–92, 1948.
20. Gregorius, F. K., Estrin, T., and Crandall, P. H.: Cervical spondylotic radiculopathy and myelopathy. Arch. Neurol. 33:618–25, 1976.
21. Stookey, B.: Compression of spinal cord and nerve roots by herniation of the nucleus pulposus in the cervical region. Arch. Surg. 40:417–32, 1940.
22. Payne, E. E. and Spillane, A. D.: The cervical spine. An anatomical-pathological study of 70 specimens. Brain 80:571–96, 1957.
23. Burrows, E. H.: The sagittal diameter of the spinal canal in cervical spondylosis. Clin. Radiol. 14:77–86, 1963.
24. Nurick, S.: The pathogenesis of the spinal cord disorder associated with cervical spondylosis. Brain 95:87–100, 1972.
25. Penning, L.: Some aspects of plain radiography of the cervical spine in chronic myelopathy. Neurology 12:513–19, 1962.
26. Bonneau, R. and Morris, J. M.: Complications of water soluble contrast lumbar myelography. Spine 3:343–5, 1970.
27. Pallis, C., Jones, A. M., and Spillane, J. D.: Cervical spondylosis. Incidence and implications. Brain 77:274–89, 1954.
28. Critchley, M.: Neurology of old age. Lancet I:1119, 1221, and 1351, 1931.
29. Howell, T. H.: Senile deterioration of central nervous system. Br. Med. J. 1:56, 1949.
30. Pearson, G. H. J.: Effect of age on vibratory sensibility. Arch. Neurol. Psychiat. 20:482, 1928.
31. Clark, E. and Robinson, P. K.: Cervical myelopathy. A complication of cervical spondylosis. Brain 79:483, 1956.
32. Crandall, P. H. and Gregorius, F. K.: Long-term follow-up of surgical treatment of cervical spondylotic myelopathy. Spine 2:139–46, 1977.

117

CHAPTER 8

Treatment: General and Specific

Whether the problems are acute or chronic, treatment of the painful neck or of problems related to the neck employs basic concepts. The intent of treating the acute problems correctly and energetically is to prevent development into the subacute and chronic conditions of pain and disability. Care of dislocation with resultant quadriplegia or of specific fractures and dislocations will only be briefly mentioned during this treatment discussion.

A careful, thorough history and physical examination are the initial steps for effective physiological treatment. The examination not only ascertains the extent and mechanism of injury but reassures the ailing patient who is usually anxious as well as in pain. Anxiety not only intensifies the pain but may aggravate many of the symptoms, compounding the difficulty in reaching a diagnosis and diminishing the patient's response to treatment.

In the acute injury, X-ray studies should be carefully reviewed for the possibility of fracture, dislocation, or both.[1, 2] With the slightest suspicion of possible fracture or dislocation, the patient should be X-rayed with extreme caution and care. The head should be maintained in neutral position with the patient in the supine position. To get a full view of all the vertebrae it may be necessary to apply gentle traction in the axial direction during the taking of the films to depress the shoulders. Ideally, a radiologist should supervise the taking of the films and review each roentgenogram as it is obtained.

When a fracture or dislocation has been ruled out, the patient should be treated conservatively. When painful limitation of movement subsides, and if symptoms so warrant, then subsequent films of the spine with the addition of full flexion and hyperextension lateral views may reveal subluxation that was not apparent in the initial X-rays.

Hospitalization in the absence of fracture or dislocation is rarely indicated unless (1) there is a history of head trauma or concussion or the history so suggests, (2) there is suspicion by the violence of the trauma or the patient's reaction that a subluxation has occurred that is not evident on preliminary examination of the X-rays, or (3) the patient's subjective complaints are so severe that ambulatory care or home care will not be satisfactory. Hospital care is valuable for the periodic observations of vital signs and for the reassurance to the extremely anxious patient by good nursing care. Traction, a cervical pillow, a collar, or merely properly positioning the patient's head and neck in this situation will usually suffice in the hospital setting, with proper medication.

Medication has definite value but definite limitations. Tranquillizers judiciously used may allay fear and act as a muscle relaxant. No drug today is totally effective as a muscle relaxant although many, by their central nervous effect, allay fear and anxiety and relax muscles that become "tensed" as a result of emotional reaction.

Excessive use of tranquillizers or sedatives is to be avoided as their action may mask important signs and symptoms and give false security to the doctor or the patient. Analgesics also are best kept at a minimum and using large doses of narcotics has the same precautions as the use of narcotics in acute head injuries or acute pain in the abdomen. These precautions need not be further clarified here.

A collar properly made and fitted and correctly used is usually beneficial. "Properly made and fitted" implies each collar being *specifically* made and fitted to the *individual* patient to hold the head and neck in a *specific position*. The slightly flexed position of the neck held within the collar is advocated as this position separates the posterior facet joints and opens the foraminae. In full flexion the spinal canal is elongated, the nerves root intradurally are elongated to a stretched position, and the ligaments and muscles of the neck are stretched with possible irritation and reflex contraction. The elongated nerve roots, by being stretched, may be stretched over an osteophytic spur or a mild herniated cervical disk.[3]

In extension (dorsiflexion) the spinal cord in the lower cervical spine becomes more slack as do the emerging nerve roots (see Chapter 1). Just as radicular pain from flexion may be caused by traction of the nerve root over a bony or disk protrusion, pain in hyperextension may result from encroachment within the foramina that are closed during extension. The clinical examination, history, and elicitation of symptoms from assuming the various positions will clarify the desired posture. With the assumption of the desired posture, symptoms of local pain and referred root pain are minimized as is nerve damage.

Using a "standard" collar with improper fitting and without subsequent evaluation is to be condemned. No two necks have a similar size or similar contour; thus, unless a collar is *specifically* fitted it may not perform the desired function and position.

No cervical orthotic device completely immobilizes the cervical spine.[4] Considered by many to be of no or very limited value, the cervical collar is still used and does give the patient subjective relief, holds the head and neck in the desired position, and restricts some motion by its contact (Fig. 86).

Neck immobilization is impossible without immobilizing the occipito-cervical articulation (occiput-atlas) and restricting movement of the atlas-axis (C_1–C_2).[5] This can be accomplished to a better degree by a "custom made" collar of felt enclosed within stockinette that wraps around the neck and includes the chin (Fig. 87). There are numerous collars made of plastic with and without metal supports or adjustments but none has proven to be more immobilizing than the

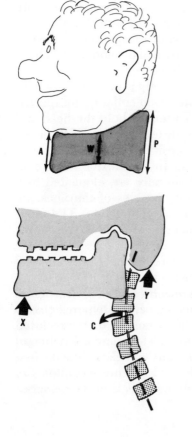

A < P

FIGURE 86. Soft cervical collar. Made of felt or similar material, the collar is narrower in the front and "supports" the chin so that the patient leans upon it thus keeping the head in a slightly flexed posture. The posterior portion is wider and acts merely as a "reminder," by contact, to prevent extension. This collar functions by kinesthetic touch rather than physical restraint or support.

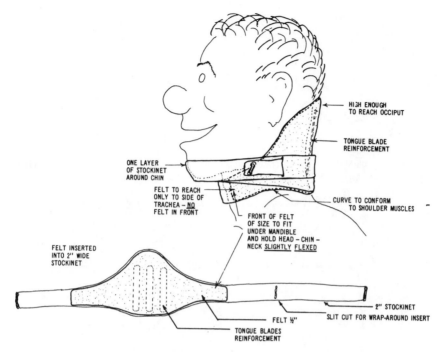

FIGURE 87. Pattern for construction of felt neck collar.

others or the felt collars. The SOMI (sternal-occipital-mandibular immobilizer) brace (Fig. 88) has recently emerged as physiologically sound, easily adjusted, and comfortably tolerated by the patient. It also has apparently been beneficial.[6]

The indications for application, time of application, and duration of wearing a collar vary with the experiences of the physician. "Early" implies application of a collar as soon as possible after the injury. This "early" may not be indicated if bed rest is chosen as the method of treatment. Even with bed rest, however, a collar may be used. If activity is contemplated, albeit with restrictions, then a collar should be applied early and continuously during periods of activity, that is, during "up" time.[7]

The collar, by encouraging a slight flexion of the cervical spine opens the foramina posteriorly, separates the zygapophyseal (facet) joints, minimizes the need for muscle "splinting," restricts excessive motion of flexion, extension, and rotation, and gives sensory cutaneous stimulation and warmth to the neck musculature which decreases pain impulses. The failure to *completely* immobilize the neck allows the muscles to contract isometrically within the confines of the collar and minimizes atrophy and disuse.

121

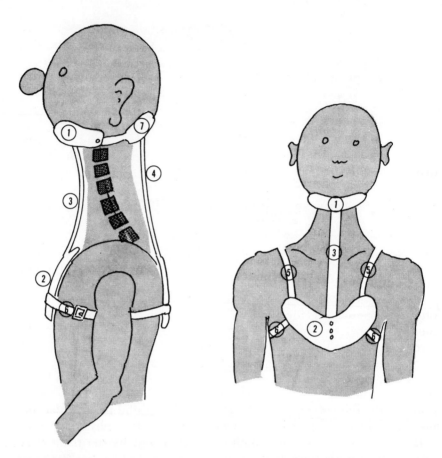

FIGURE 88. SOMI cervical orthosis. This brace is molded with plastic and metal to conform to portions of the head and the shoulders. It fits under the chin (1), and holds the submandibular portion in place by a bent vertical bar (3) arising from a pad against the sternum (2). A posterior bar (4) supports the occipital pad (7). Straps (5), (6), (7) fasten the brace to the body and pass over the shoulders.

From the first day to a minimum (usually) of one week the collar can be worn continuously during the day when awake and upright, gradually being decreased to wearing intermittently, and then after 10 to 14 days[8] worn only when riding in a car, when fatigued or when an activity is required that may make it difficult to observe or maintain correct posture.

Splinting should *not* be prolonged. To maintain a collar for an excessive period of time (in excess of two weeks in the usual acute injury) will lead to (1) muscular disuse atrophy, (2) fibrous contracture from organization of the accumulated edema, (3) shortening of the sustained contracted muscles, (4) thickening of the facet capsular tissues, and (5) increased dependency enhancing neurosis or extension of traumatic neurosis.[9]

Toward the end of the first week, gentle activities during brief periods out of the collar are begun. A "chin in" posture is taught and while in this position gentle progressive rotation to the left and to the right are initiated. *Flexion and extension are to be avoided.* Removal of the collar should be gradual but progressive so that by the second week the patient need wear the collar only while driving or being driven in a car, when performing strenuous activities, or when tired or under duress. During these activities, the collar protects against untoward movements, prevents sustained positions considered undesirable, and keeps the neck warm and thus comfortable and relaxed. Some patients cannot tolerate a collar for various reasons. Whatever the reason, be it physical discomfort or psychological reasons, there should be no insistence upon its being worn as it may nullify any benefit desired.

For sleep or for lying in the supine position, a cervical pillow is often comfortable for the patient (Fig. 89). There are numerous commercial brands and designs but most are shaped to fill in the cervical lordosis to a degree yet support the head at the occiput to maintain slight neck flexion. The pillow also "cradles" the head on each side to prevent lateral flexion and rotation. Sleeping with a cervical collar is not well tolerated by some patients and does not provide lateral support to prevent patients from lying on their sides. The pillow supplements daytime wearing of the collar.

Heat applied in its many forms is advocated by many. Excessive heat tends to aggravate muscle spasm and intensify pain in the early phase of treatment. Warmth is well tolerated and is soothing. This can

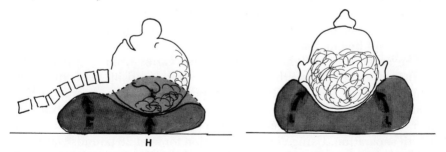

H

FIGURE 89. Cervical pillow. There are numerous commercial brands and designs but most are shaped to fill in the cervical lordosis (C) to a degree yet support the head (H) at the occiput to maintain slight neck flexion. The pillow also "cradles" the head on each side to prevent lateral flexion and rotation (L).

be administered in the home by an electric heating pad at the low temperature, a warm shower, warm moist towels, or a 100 watt light bulb placed two feet away. Stronger heat for longer periods is of value later when active exercises are added to increase the range of motion.

Initially, after the injury, the application of ice packs is well worth trying. If tolerated, it can be very soothing and relieve pain. Ice cubes chipped finely, held in a plastic pack covered with a towel, then wrapped around the posteriolateral aspect of the neck and held for 15 to 20 minutes is effective. Ice tends to (1) decongest the superficial tissues, (2) be analgesic, and (3) act upon the spindle cells of the muscles to effect muscular relaxation.

During the early period of recovery, the frequent "office or clinic visit" for the mere application of heat, be it diathermy, ultrasound, or other modalities, is inadvisable. The travel time, the discomfort and anxiety of traveling, the usual delay in the waiting room, and so forth, all nullify any possible benefit from the treatment proffered there.

Massage is valuable for its sedative effect and its dissipation action on accumulated fluids. Circulation is also enhanced. Here, too, benefits are derived *after* the acute phase is passed. At the onset, the tissues are usually too sensitive for any effective massage, and no position is possible during the massage that permits total relaxation of the patient.

Medical literature is replete with articles on the efficacy of cervical traction.[10] Only personal experience determines the method, the amount of weight applied, the duration, and the frequency of traction, since, unfortunately, no scientific documentation is available. Only the *position of the neck during traction* is generally accepted.

Cervical traction effects its benefits by *immobilizing* the neck when it is used in a *continuous* manner from a *reclining* position. When used intermittently traction functions by *elongating* the neck and *straightening* the cervical *lordosis*. This position of slight flexion opens the posterior articulations, widens the intervertebral foramina, disengages the facet surfaces, and elongates the posterior muscular tissues and ligaments. The effect of traction on the disks is debated.

The amount of weight or traction pull varies from one pound to sufficient weight to lift the patient completely off his feet. In a laboratory study,[11] a traction force of 260 pounds caused a separation of 2 mm between vertebrae C_5–C_6 and C_6–C_7. Manual traction estimated to be 300 pounds[12] allegedly doubles the intervertebral spaces in width separation. Using vertebral traction force of 25 pounds was considered the minimum that would straighten the cervical lordosis.[13] Studies of force and the angle of traction[14-16] indicate that a traction pull of 30 pounds separates the vertebrae posteriorly. The greater the posterior separation with the greatest foraminal opening occurs at a degree angle of 24°.

The duration of traction is arbitrary but the amount of traction is that which is tolerated by the patient and benefits the patient's problem. Obviously the intent of traction is the *decrease of the lordosis and not distraction of the offending functional unit.* Application of traction in slight flexion accomplishes the same separation with less force and thus with less discomfort experienced by the patient.

In a controlled series of several hundred patients treated with cervical traction,[17] patients with radiculopathy (pain and tingling radiating down to the hand and fingers) benefited the most. Patients complaining of headaches in the frontal area or occipital region benefited the least. There was no explanation for these conclusions.

Cervical traction may be applied in one of three ways: (1) reclining traction (Figs. 90 and 91) beginning with 5 pounds for 30 minutes daily and increasing the weight in increments of 2 to 3 pounds daily until 25 to 30 pounds is reached, (2) full body weight traction from the sitting position (Fig. 92) for periods of 5 minutes daily (the proper seated position must be carefully observed here; this type of traction is best administered at first in the office until the manner is judged to be correct and the patient does not experience fear or resistance), or (3) mechanical motorized intermittent traction. This last type of traction can be applied in the seated or the supine position and has a massagelike effect that is better tolerated than fixed traction. The disadvantage is that the patient must make office visits rather than treat himself at home; and since home treatment can be more frequent, it can be more effective. Intermittent traction may not be tolerated by patients who have acute pain with "irritable" muscles. The undulating traction apparently initiates a stretch reflex by elongating the muscle fibril and the spindle-Golgi apparatus. This being done repeatedly may not allow the muscle to "unload" and relax. Relaxation and elongation of the muscle fibers does not result and the benefit of traction is not achieved.

The method of attaching any form of traction to the head remains a source of concern since no halter is effective or comfortable. As shown in Figure 93, there is little posterior prominence upon which to attach and lift, and the anterior point of attachment, the mandible, transmits much of its pull through the dentures and the temporomandibular joint, both potentially painful areas. The long anterior lever arm versus the shorter rear one has the effect of causing extension of the neck rather than the desired flexion. This is combatted by having the line of pull "up and forward" and placing the patient so as to "lie back into the sling." The "slumped" position must be accompanied by *total body relaxation.*

A commonly prescribed home traction is by a door attachment in which the door is used against which to apply traction or a bag, usually filled with water, is the applied traction. This form of traction is not

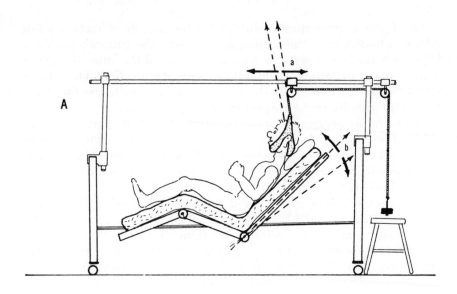

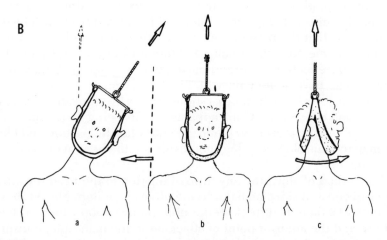

FIGURE 90. Bed cervical traction, hospital type. *A,* The patient should be seated in a slightly flexed position with hips and knees flexed and low back relaxed. The traction should come from above and ahead of the trunk. Pulley *a* may be moved ahead or behind to alter direction of traction. The neck, however, should always be flexed. The line of pull may be altered by changing inclination of the bed, *b.* A stool should be under the weights so that the distance is very short in case of a sudden drop or fall. The stool is also convenient for the periods during which the traction is released. A monkey bar may be hung from the overhead bar for the patient's convenience. *B,* The manner of direct traction with head straight ahead, *b,* and with head rotated, *c.* By laterally shifting the body, *a,* the traction causes lateral stretch as well as direct traction.

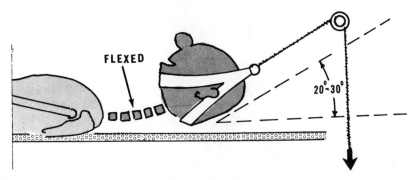

FIGURE 91. Cervical traction applied to the supine patient causing cervical spine flexion with the angle of pull between 20 and 30 degrees.

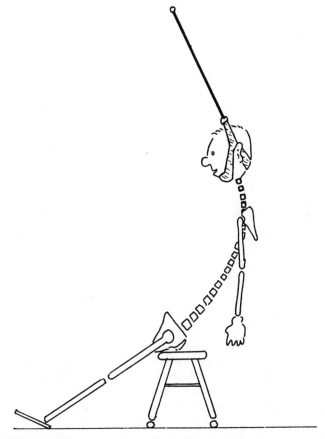

FIGURE 92. Overhead cervical traction for home use. With the rope securely fastened overhead and slightly in front of the seated patient, the traction is applied on the flexed neck. The patient should be seated in a fully relaxed position with low back flexed, legs extended, and arms dangling at his side. This position attains maximum relaxation.

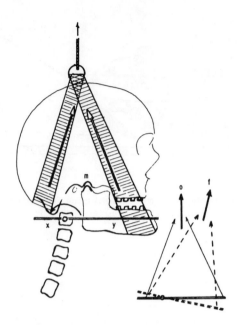

FIGURE 93. Angle of traction on head halter. The head halter superimposed upon the skull depicts the short lever arm and small point of attachment at the base of the skull, x, and the longer lever arm under the chin at y. If traction is from direction o, the longer arm would tend to extend the neck; but by advancing the traction above and ahead of the head, the direction of pull tends to cause neck flexion. It is evident that the pressure from traction arm y is concentrated on the teeth and at the temporomandibular joint, m.

favored by the author. The door must be kept unlocked to permit the overhead attachment to be inserted; thus, the traction equipment is unstable. If the water bag is used, it is bulky and awkward. It mandates filling and emptying the bag with water, the weight never varies, and any mishap poses a housekeeping problem. Also, it is difficult for the patient to face the door and extend his legs fully and maintain the desired 20 to 25° flexion traction angle (Fig. 94).

In the absence of fracture dislocation *forceful traction in the early phase of an acute neck injury should be avoided.* Forceful traction in this condition is pitted against spasm that is splinting acutely inflamed tissues. Elongation of these irritated tissues can only injure them further. Traction for reduction of a fracture or dislocation is another instance in which traction *must* overcome spasm.

During the early recovery period when active range of motion becomes desirable, traction is best applied *manually,* concomitantly with exercise. Manual traction has the advantage of greater control of the position of the head and individual grading of the amount and duration of traction.

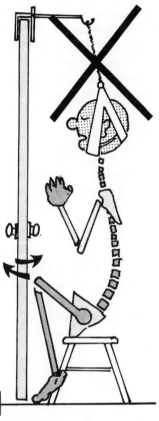

FIGURE 94. Ineffective home door cervical traction. The patient is too close to the door to get the correct neck flexion angle. The door freely opens and closes, not permitting constant traction. The patient cannot extend the legs or assume a comfortable position. This type of home traction is not recommended.

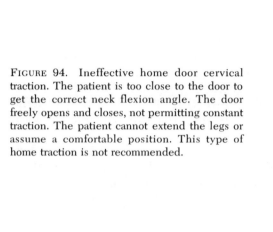

Occasionally there is segmental limitation and restriction of motion of the cervical spine at a specific level. This is not easily determined and requires years of practice and careful evaluation.

The exact mechanism for this segmental motion limitation has been attributed to a "locked zygapophyseal joint," a segmental contracture after a mild segmental subluxation, or merely "minor joint dysfunction." Local pain can be attributed to periarticular inflammation of the facet joint and referred pain attributed to inflammation or entrapment of a contiguous nerve root.

Examination requires careful segmental passive range of motion of each joint with the patient supine as well as with the patient seated. In the supine position, there is greater ease of relaxation of the patient's neck muscles and a greater passive range of motion due to elimination of gravity. These two factors decrease the cervical lordosis. Relaxation of the patient also is enhanced.

The examiner can *manually* apply gentle traction, lateral flexion to either side, and with careful placement of the hands can determine the passive range at almost each cervical segment. Rotation can also be evaluated and its level determined. The degree of passive range limitation, with or without pain being elicited by that specific movement, can be recorded in the manner described by Maigne[18] (Fig. 95).

Recording subsequent examinations in this way can determine increase or decrease in range and change in pain in that particular direction. By this method, progress can also be recorded as related to specific therapy.

A particularly painful segment (functional unit) can be specified by precise manual examination. Movement of the vertebral body by direct pressure upon the posterior superior spinous process can designate the specific site of pain. Lateral movement of the vertebra as is possible at the thoracic or lumbar level (Fig. 96) is more difficult at the cervical level. The zygapophyseal joints are easily palpable and local tenderness can be elicited.

Finding the segmental limitation of movement and localized tenderness will frequently identify the site of local neck pain or the site of origin of referred root pain. Manipulation of the specifically involved joint has been advocated by many[18-20] as effective when other forms of treatment have failed.

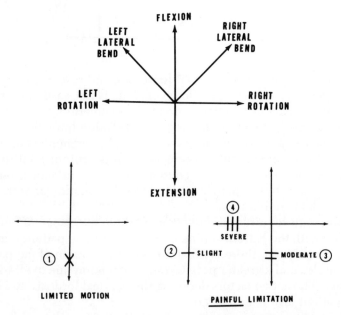

FIGURE 95. Recording of range of motion of cervical spine. Lines are used to indicate restriction and simultaneous pain, and X is used to indicate mere limitation and no pain.

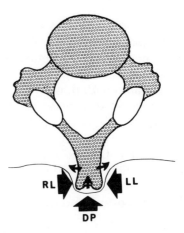

FIGURE 96. Methods of movement of the vertebral segment with direct pressure (*DP*) or right lateral (*RL*) or left lateral (*LL*) pressure upon the posterior superior spine.

Maigne[18] has advocated moving the involved joint segment in the direction *opposite* to that of restriction or pain. This painless, free moving range of motion rather than attempting to overcome limitation by forcing the joint in the direction of resistance is claimed to accomplish the desired increase.

Finding a specific zygapophyseal joint tenderness also localizes a painful joint that is amenable to intra-articular injection of a local anesthetic and steroid. Such an injection, with proper localization and proper technique, is safe and reasonably easily performed.

Adjunctive treatment preceding traction may consist of hot, moist packs, ethyl chloride spray, massage, or injections of "trigger points" with procaine. Ethyl chloride spray probably works on a reflex counterirritant basis and must be applied by a person fully aware of the precise method of application and its possible dangers. Injecting painful areas with an anesthetic can be dramatic not only in permitting traction but in relieving pain. The sites of injection are usually at the points of deep tenderness and can be ascertained by the pain being temporarily initiated or aggravated during the administration of the injection.

In a trial program of treatment[21] to compare the various modalities of traction, collar, posture, placebo, and short wave diathermy, only the diathermy was the placebo modality. The conclusions were of interest:

1. The rate of improvement was essentially identical in all varied groups.
2. Assuming the position of the traction was as effective as the application of traction.
3. Posture training was as effective as a collar and/or traction.

131

Factors affecting the end result were age, initial severity of the attack, and the number of previous attacks. There was no significant difference noted in patients with objective neurological signs as compared with those without, or in patients with limited range of motion as compared with those without. Carefully controlled studies such as this are needed to evaluate the efficacy of all treatment modalities.

Exercises begin in the second phase of treatment. The objective of exercise is to elongate the soft tissues to their normal range, minimize periarticular fibrous contracture of the zygapophyseal joints, regain the normal length of muscle, and, by muscular action, to increase circulation to the deep neck tissues. By improving flexibility and muscle tone, posture and neck function can be improved.

An extremely effective form of exercise is the *active-assisted-resisted* method termed *rhythmic stabilization*.[22, 23] This exercise accomplishes all the physiological effects of exercise just listed. It does so in a safe, progressive, and well tolerated manner. The technique must be learned by the patient and by the therapist (Fig. 97).

In essence, the exercise is movement of the patient's neck by the therapist, which is resisted by the patient so that no movement, but merely muscle contraction (isometric contraction), results. Firmly holding the patient's slightly flexed head in both hands, the therapist begins a slow, gradual lateral movement of the head. The force by the therapist undulates slowly from slight to strong to slight pressure, and it is resisted by *equal* force by the patient. No movement occurs, and there are no abrupt, jerky muscle contractions. Each contraction is followed by a rest period during which blood flows into the muscle. Each cycle of exercise is done at a different degree of lateral flexion and rotation. Ultimately a full range of motion is attained.

Once the acute condition has completely abated, as evidenced by an absence of symptoms, negative physical findings, full range of motion, and no functional limitation, the patient should be instructed in range of motion exercises to retain flexibility and advised regarding proper total body posture and proper position of the neck during everyday activities.

Proper posture and proper use of the neck follow a few basic concepts: *Avoid any prolonged position. Maintain mobility. Avoid acute or prolonged extension* of the neck. *Minimize prolonged hyperflexion.* For good posture, *maintain flat neck* attitude: chin in, head up, and head back (Fig. 98).

The present use of car seat belts neither prevents nor diminishes deceleration accidents with hyperflexion or hyperextension injuries to the neck. In fact, by securing the lower portion of the body to the car, it is conceivable that the "whiplash" effect *to the neck* is enhanced. The present high rolled pillow extending above the back of the seat

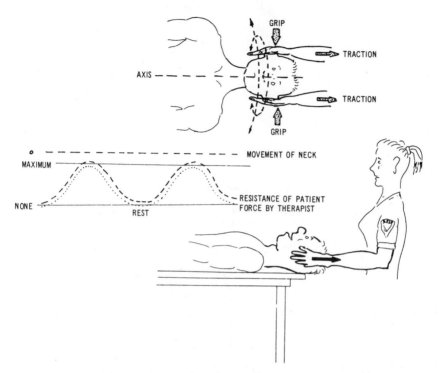

FIGURE 97. Rhythmic stabilization exercises to neck. This active, assisted exercise should be applied by a trained person. The traction is applied manually in the line of the neck, preferably with the head more elevated than shown here, so that the neck is slightly flexed. As the therapist moves the patient's head to the side (lateral flexion) or attempts rotation of the head, the patient resists with the exact pressure as applied by the therapist so that no movement occurs. Movement is rhythmically attempted, and the degree of lateral flexion and/or rotation is altered after several cycles. See text.

and fitted to the level of the back of the head appears to be a step in the right direction. Automotive engineers working with medical authorities have a significant challenge here.

Last, but not least, in the treatment of the cervical sprain syndrome, especially when there is a preponderance of bizarre symptoms that defy plausible explanation, an excess of emotional tension effect, and an undue prolongation of disability from the symptoms, attention must be paid to the psychogenic aspects of the illness. Unfortunately such symptoms are frequently interpreted as malingering. This is especially true when much of the "symptomatology disappears after legal settlement."[24] The patient frequently considers the stress of litigation, with the prolonging of investigations and repeated medical examinations culminating in unpleasant court appearances, to be "more

133

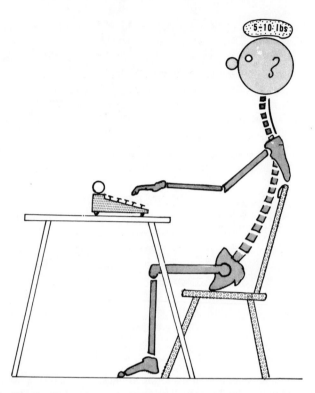

FIGURE 98. Distraction exercise for posture training. With a weight of 5 to 10 pounds within a sandbag upon the head, the posture is maintained erect and the cervical lordosis is minimal. Proprioceptive concept of posture is learned with no effort.

traumatic than was the injury," and he often welcomes settlement even when it is unrewarding financially.

The anxiety resulting from a cervical injury is often not allayed by adequate reassurance from the doctor. Haphazard treatment may fail to afford relief and may leave the patient impressed with "a serious injury that is not responding to treatment." Such a threat to security may well psychologically decompensate a previously tense, emotionally unstable person, or one who has personality aberrations. Evidence of psychological abnormality should be recognized immediately and adequate treatment instituted, be it reassurance, drug therapy, or psychotherapy.

When should the physician resort to surgery? No time factor is used in deciding on this question unless the impatience and social-economic aspect of the patient's disability enter the picture. The true indications for surgery should be considered very carefully as *a last resort* when (1) exhaustive conservative treatment has failed, (2) in spite of conservative treatment, there is evidence of progressive neurological deficit, (3) long tract signs attributable to cervical pathology exist, (4) diagnostic studies have ruled out other pathological states and reasonably ascertain cervical causative factors, (5) the definite symptomatic level has been determined, and (6) the specific surgical approach has been ascertained and the qualifications and limitations of the surgeon have been recognized.

Surgical procedures vary from laminotomy and diskectomy, laminectomy with dentate ligament section for decompression, to a combination of both of these and simultaneous fusion. Interbody fusion from an anterior approach is advocated by many surgical centers because (1) the approach is more direct to the disk and avoids injury to the spinal cord and nerve roots, (2) the procedure is technically not difficult, (3) the disk and/or the posterior osteophyte can be removed, (4) all cervical levels between C_2 and C_7 can be visualized, (5) any vertebral dislocation can be reduced under direct visualization, and (6) the hospital sojourn is markedly reduced since ambulation is early. In the posterior approach, when a laminectomy is performed later, posterior fusion is difficult and even impossible. The decision of *fusion or no fusion* is still an unresolved surgical question.

REFERENCES

1. Charlton, O. P., Gehweiler, J. A. and Martinez, S.: Roentgenographic evaluation of cervical spine trauma. J.A.M.A. 242:1073–5, 1978.
2. Miller, M. D., et al.: Significant new observations in cervical spine trauma. Am. J. Roentgenol. 130:659–63, 1978.
3. Fisher, S. V., et al.: Cervical orthosis effect on cervical spine motion: Roentgenographic and goniometric method of study. Arch. Phys. Med. Rehabil. 58:109–15, 1977.
4. Jones, M. D.: Cineradiographic studies of collar-immobilized cervical spine. J. Neurosurg. 17:633–7, 1960.
5. Jones, M. D.: Cineradiologic studies of the normal cervical spine. Calif. Med. 93:293–6, 1960.
6. Hartman, J. T., Palumbo, F., and Hill, B. J.: Cineradiography of braced normal cervical spine: Comparative study of five commonly used cervical orthosis. Clin. Orthop. 109:97–102, 1975.
7. Gay, J. R. and Abbott, K. H.: Common whiplash injuries of the neck. J.A.M.A. 127:1698–704, 1953.
8. Symonds, C.: The inter-relation of trauma and cervical spondylosis in compression of the cervical cord. Lancet 1:451, 1953.
9. Eastwood, W. J. and Jefferson, G.: Discussion on fractures and dislocation of the cervical vertebrae. Proc. R. Soc. Med. 33:651–60, 1940.
10. Caldwell, J. W. and Krusen, E. M.: Effectiveness of cervical traction in treatment of neck problems: Evaluations of various methods. Arch. Phys. Med. Rehabil. 43:214–21, 1962.
11. DeSeze, and Levernieux, J.: Les traction vertebrales: Premiere etud experimentales et resultats therapeutique d'apres une experience de quatres annees. Semaine des Hopitaux (de Paris) 27:2085–104, 1951.

12. Cyriax, J.: Textbook of Orthopedic Medicine, ed. 4, vol. 1: Diagnosis of soft tissue lesions. New York, Harper & Row, 1962, pp. 171–2.
13. Judavitch, B. D.: Herniated cervical disc: A new form of traction therapy. Am. J. Surg. 84:646–56, 1962.
14. Colachis, S. C. and Strohm, B. R.: A study of tractive forces and angle of pull on vertebral interspaces in the cervical spine. Arch. Phys. Med. Rehabil. 46:820–30, 1965.
15. Colachis, S. C. and Strohm, B. R.: Cervical traction: Relationship of traction time to varied traction forces with constant angle of pull. Arch. Phys. Med. Rehabil. 46:815–9, 1965.
16. Colachis S. C. and Strohm, B. R.: Radiographic studies of cervical spine motion in normal subjects: Flexion and hyperextension. Arch. Phys. Med. Rehabil. 46:753–60, 1965.
17. Valtowen, E. J. and Kiuro, E.: Cervical traction as a therapeutic tool. Scand. J. Rehabil. Med. 2:29–36, 1970.
18. Maigne, R.: Orthopedic Medicine. Springfield, Ill., Charles C Thomas, 1972.
19. Bourdillion, J. F.: Spinal Manipulation. New York, Appleton-Century-Crofts, 1970.
20. Mennell, J.: Treatment by Movement and Massage, ed. 5. London, Churchill, 1945.
21. Pain in the neck and arm: A multicentre trial of the effects of physiotherapy. Br. Med. J. 29:254–8, 1966.
22. Rubin, D.: Head, neck, and arm symptoms subsequent to neck injuries: Physical therapeutic considerations. Arch. Phys. Med. Rehabil. 40:387–9, 1959.
23. Kabat, H.: Central facilitation: The basis of treatment for paralysis. Permanente Found. Med. Bull. 10:190–204, 1952.
24. Frankel, C. J.: Medical-legal aspects of injuries to the neck. J.A.M.A. 169:216–23, 1959.

136

CHAPTER 9

Differential Diagnosis

Many conditions simulate pain in the neck and the shoulder and feelings of discomfort and dysasthesias in the upper extremity that must be differentiated as to their origin and mechanism of production. Symptoms presented are similar to those of the local neck pain, and the peripheral symptoms resemble those that have been attributed to conditions of nerves and blood vessels encroached upon from inadequate space or abnormal movement in the neck.

The "compression syndromes" that mimic peripheral neuropathic conditions include the scalene anticus syndrome, the claviculocostal syndrome, and the pectoralis minor syndrome. All three of these syndromes have one common denominator: their symptoms and signs are attributed to *compression of the neurovascular bundle in the region of the cervical thoracic dorsal outlet.* The neurovascular bundle is the grouping of the brachial plexus nerve fibers and the subclavian artery and vein. It is located in the region of the apex of the rib cage (the cervical-dorsal outlet) bounded medially by the first rib, anteriorly by the upper portion of the sternum, and posteriorly by the first thoracic vertebra.

The brachial plexus (Fig. 99) is composed of the primary anterior rami[1] of C_5, C_6, C_7, C_8, and T_1. The rami (roots) emerging from the intervertebral foramen are situated between the scalene muscles. As they proceed laterally and downward, they merge into three trunks (upper C_5 and C_6, middle C_7, lower C_8 and T_1). The trunks are located in the supraclavicular fossa just lateral to the scalene muscles. The trunks divide and pass under the clavicle just lateral to the first rib. The divisions unite to form the cords located in the axilla. These three cords give rise to the majority of the peripheral nerves of the upper extremities.

The subclavian artery arches over the first rib and there joins the brachial plexus just behind the insertion site of the anterior scalene

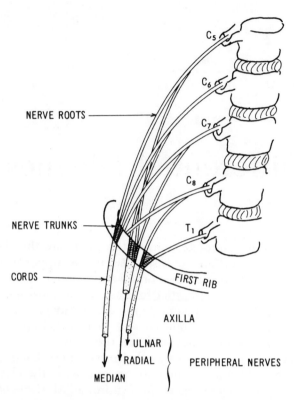

NERVE ROOTS

C_5

C_6

C_7

C_8

T_1

NERVE TRUNKS

FIRST RIB

CORDS

AXILLA

ULNAR

RADIAL

PERIPHERAL NERVES

MEDIAN

FIGURE 99.   Brachial plexus (schematic). The brachial plexus is composed of the anterior primary rami of segments C_5, C_6, C_7, C_8, and T_1. The *roots* emerge from the intervertebral foramina through the *scalene muscles*. The roots merge into three *trunks* in the region of the first rib. The trunks via divisions become *cords* that divide into the peripheral nerves of the upper extremities.

muscle (Fig. 100). The subclavian vein is anterior medial to the subclavian artery and is separated from it by the anterior scalene muscle.

The pain syndromes of the cervical dorsal outlet are essentially compression symptoms of the neurovascular bundle as it passes over and past the first rib or of the nerve portion of the bundle as it (brachial plexus) emerges and proceeds forward and downward from the groove of the transverse process.

The symptoms vary depending upon whether the nerves, the blood vessels, or both are compressed. Nerve compression symptoms are the most frequent and consist of paresthesia, pain, and subjective weakness.

The distribution of pain can be insidious and can include the neck, shoulder, arm, or hand. Most frequently the symptoms are paresthesia of ulnar nerve distribution.

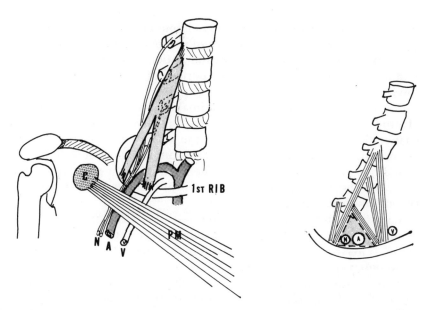

FIGURE 100. The supraclavicular space. The scalene muscles originate from the cervical spine and divide to contain the brachial plexus (N) and the subclavian artery (A). The middle scalene muscle is posterior and the anterior scalene muscle is anterior to the artery. The subclavian vein (V) is anterior to the anterior scalene muscle. After passing over the first rib (not shown) the neurovascular bundle passes under the smaller pectoral muscle. The clavicle covers the neurovascular bundle and lies parallel to the first rib. The coracoid process is labeled C.

Vascular symptoms may be arterial or venous and vary from Raynaud's phenomenon to edema, pallor, venous congestion, and discoloration. The loss or decrease of palpable pulsations is described in subsequent pages regarding various diagnostic maneuvers.

Clinically the findings may be sparce but there has been great credence to verification of the syndrome by the prolongation of the ulnar nerve conduction velocity (UNCV).[2] Nerve conduction velocities are performed to determine decrease of velocity at the first rib level of the brachial plexus. The nerve is stimulated at the supraclavicular fossa, the middle of the upper arm, and between the elbow and the hand, and is picked up at the hypothenar eminence. Prolonged velocities across the outlet can be determined and are diagnostic.

ANTERIOR SCALENE SYNDROME

Symptoms of the anterior scalene syndrome[3, 4] are *numbness* and *tingling* ("going to sleep" or "pins and needles" feeling) of the arm, hand, and fingers, diminished sensation, and weakness of finger movements and grip. Pain is usually claimed to be a deep, dull, vague "aching" in the arm and hand. All of these symptoms appear during early morning hours and awaken the patient, or they come on after prolonged sitting or after extended periods of seated activities such as sewing or knitting.

Physical findings are usually minimal or absent. Objective changes of atrophy, reflex loss, swelling of the supraclavicular area, and trophic changes (color changes, coldness of the hand, excessive perspiration) are usually absent. Some equivocal pin prick sensation or light touch sensations may be felt as "less." The findings are essentially subjective, and the examination is that of reproducing the symptoms by specific motions and positions.

A positive diagnostic test is the so-called "Adson Test," which would best be termed Scalene Anticus Test rather than by a proper name. This test consists of turning the head *to* the side of the symptoms, *extending* the head (backwards), abducting the arm, taking a deep breath, and obliterating the radial pulse *in that arm* and *reduplicating the symptoms complained of* by the patient.

The mechanism causing these symptoms and which is reproduced in the test is as follows: The anterior scalene muscles originate from the transverse processes of the third through the sixth cervical vertebrae. They insert in a broad band into the upper surface of the first rib near the sternum; and as the brachial plexus and the subclavian artery pass over the rib, the latter pass in an angle formed by the scalene insertion to the rib (Fig. 101). The Adson test maneuver theoretically contracts the scalene muscle and narrows the angle (by rotation and extension) and elevates the rib (by the deep breath—the scalene being an accessory deep inspiratory muscle). The effects on the neurovascular bundle are those of traction and mostly compression.

Why these symptoms should occur, usually in later life, is theoretical. The *spasm* of the scalene muscles may result from fatigue from unusual exercise or physical activity. Trauma from a deceleration hyperextension accident may have been causative. A significant change in posture as a result of an illness, an emotional strain, or an occupational period of stress may well stress the scalenes. All too often no etiological factors are discovered in taking the history.

The most plausible cause of scalene *spasm*[5] is nerve root irritation in the region of the intervertebral foramina. This is the mechanism depicted in Figure 23, with the muscle spasm being a reflex phenomenon regardless of the type of nerve root irritation. The most probable irritation to the nerve in this age group would be cervical spondylosis or zygapophyseal joint inflammation intruding into the foramen.

It has been postulated that the nerve roots are compressed by the scalene muscles where the muscular origin from the transverse proc-

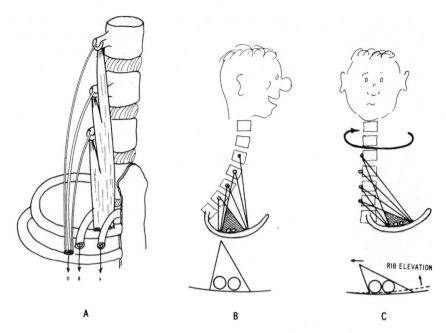

A   B   C

FIGURE 101. Scalene anticus syndrome. *A*, Relationship of the neurovascular bundle. The subclavian artery, *a*, passes behind the anterior scalene muscle, loops over the first rib, and is joined by the brachial plexus, *n*. The artery is separated from the subclavian vein, *v*, by the anterior scalene muscle. The median scalene muscle (not shown) lies behind the nerve *n*. *B*, The triangle formed by the scalenes and the first rib. *C*, Distortion from turning the head toward the symptomatic side. Also, the first rib elevates as a result of deep inspiration, the scalenes being inspiratory muscles. Compression of the neurovascular bundle *n*, *a*, and occasionally *v* can be pictured from the test maneuver of the anticus scalene syndrome.

ess "pinches" the nerve one level below between it and the lower bony process. The brachial plexus roots pass close to the origins of the scalene muscles, but the transverse processes separate the muscle bellies and make "scissoring" improbable.

The presence of a cervical rib or a large transverse process of C_7 has been implicated in the etiology of the scalene anticus syndrome. Pressure from the rib or the rib as an aberrant site of scalene muscle attachment has been blamed for compressing the neurovascular bundle. This is highly improbable, since the cervical rib has been present for a lifetime without causing trouble. Also, its removal frequently does not afford relief. Most patients with cervical ribs have no symptoms, and most patients with symptoms have no cervical ribs. The cervical rib, therefore, is responsible in very few instances, and *its removal should be delayed until all else is tried.*

Treatment of the anticus scalene syndrome is similar to the treatment of the cervical diskogenic syndrome, namely, improving flexi-

141

bility and improving posture by decreasing the cervical lordosis, thus opening the posterior foramina, the means of doing this being exercises, traction, collar, muscle-relaxant drugs, and posture training. Injection of the scalene muscles with novocaine or resection of the scalene muscles surgically probably has value by releasing pressure upon the cervical spine.

As many of the patients with cervical dorsal outlet syndrome are middle-aged and demonstrate weakness and fatigue of the shoulder girdle muscles, exercises to strengthen these muscles are valuable.

"Shrugging" (scapular elevation) against resistance, for strength, range of motion, and endurance will benefit this type of patient. Posture will also be benefited by means of these exercises as well as opening the cervical dorsal outlet. In the seated position, with the neck in a decreased lordotic posture, the shoulders are elevated slowly, repeatedly, and fully against increasing resistance and with increasing repetitions (Fig. 102). The same exercise is also performed

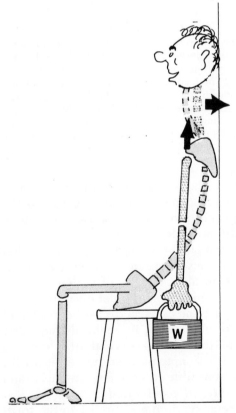

FIGURE 102. Posture-scapular elevation exercises. Patient is seated with back to wall, his head and neck pressed against the wall, which decreases the cervical lordosis. With arms fully extended and dependent, weights are lifted in a shrugging motion. Weights vary from 5 to 30 pounds.

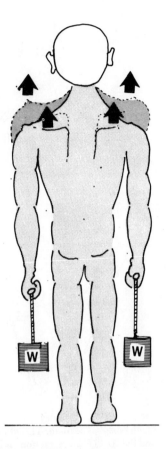

FIGURE 103. Standing scapular elevation exercises. With proper posture (tilted pelvis and flattened cervical lordosis) both arms are rhythmically elevated, held, and slowly lowered. Increasing weights are used. Elbows must be fully extended.

in the standing position, making sure that the shoulders are elevated and posteriorly retracted and that the posture (decreased cervical and lumbar lordosis) be properly maintained (Fig. 103).

In determining the cause of the symptoms of anticus syndrome, it is always prudent to consider the syndrome as a *secondary* condition resulting from, possibly, radiculitis of a cervical root, inflammatory lesion of the cervical spine, interspinous lesion, or even a referred syndrome from the pericardium or diaphragm. The syndrome may be secondary to shoulder pericapsulitis, which will be discussed later in this chapter.

CLAVICULOCOSTAL SYNDROME

Symptoms of neurovascular compression can occur from pressure on the bundle between the first rib and the clavicle[6] (claviculocostal) at the point where the brachial plexus joins the supraclavicular artery and courses over the first rib (Fig. 104).

143

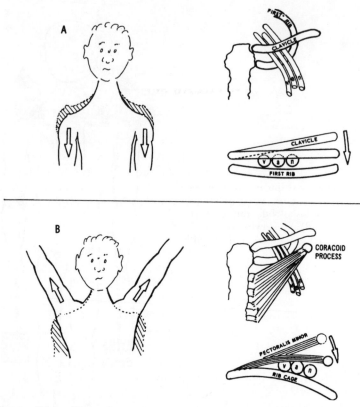

FIGURE 104. Claviculocostal syndrome and pectoralis minor syndrome. A, Claviculocostal syndrome. The neurovascular bundle is compressed between the clavicle and the first rib by retraction and depression of the shoulder girdles. B, Pectoralis minor syndrome. The neurovascular bundle may be compressed between the pectoralis minor and the rib cage by elevating the arms in a position of abduction and moving the arms behind the head.

The same etiological factors of fatigue, trauma, and postural changes enter here also, and an *a*symmetrical thoracic outlet is frequently found on X-ray. The symptoms are paresthesia, numbness, and/or pain in the arm and hand chiefly at night or in the early morning. Trophic changes, atrophy, reflex changes, and weakness may be present, but as a rule the findings and the symptoms are transient.

The diagnosis is made by *simultaneously obliterating the radial pulse and reduplicating the symptoms* by bringing the shoulders back and down—actively by the patient—then, passively, with some pressure by the examiner.

The treatment here is postural improvement, increase in neck flexibility, and improvement of the muscle tone of the shoulder girdles.

144

Emotional factors—especially depression—which permit slumping and "picturing of a fatigue state" must be appreciated, and treatment must be undertaken in this direction.

PECTORALIS MINOR SYNDROME
(HYPERABDUCTION SYNDROME)

The pectoralis minor muscles originate from the third, fourth, and fifth ribs (occasionally the second and sixth) in the anterior midcostal area and insert into the coracoid process of the scapula. As the brachial plexus (the cord division) descends over the rib cage in the axilla, accompanied by the axillary vein and artery (the continuation of the subclavian artery), it is covered by the pectoralis minor. The vascular compression syndrome occurs supposedly from compression of the bundle between the pectoralis minor and the rib cage (Fig. 104).

The symptoms are identical to those of the claviculocostal compression syndrome, are transient and usually *un*accompanied by objective changes, and occur during the night or early morning.

The diagnostic feature is the *obliteration of the radial pulse and reduplication of the symptoms* by bringing the arms overhead, abducted, and slightly backward. This is a maneuver that places the pectoralis minor on stretch. The treatment should correct the (usual) slumped posture, stretch the pectoral muscles, correct the habit or occupational slumped posture, and combat any effect of depression or emotional tension on posture.

SCAPULOCOSTAL SYNDROME

As has been stated, pain referred from cervical diskogenic nerve root irritation can be referred to the interscapular region especially to the supermedial angle of the scapula, and a musculoskeletal complex causing pain must be differentiated in the diagnostic consideration of neck-shoulder pain.

The so-called scapulocostal syndrome (Fig. 105) is musculoskeletal pain,[7] a myofascial-periosteal strain with local tenderness and pain at the site of insertion of the levator scapulae muscles to the scapula. The etiology is usually postural, whether from such physical causes as overexertion, prolonged occupational postural stress, or fatigue, or from emotional stress that causes myostatic tension or slumped, "weight-of-the-world-on-my-shoulders" posture, or from a tense, hostile, aggressive attitude that affects the posture. There are no neurological signs or symptoms.

The treatment is a mechanical release of muscular tension by a "figure 8" shoulder harness for a week to 10 days, anti-inflammatory

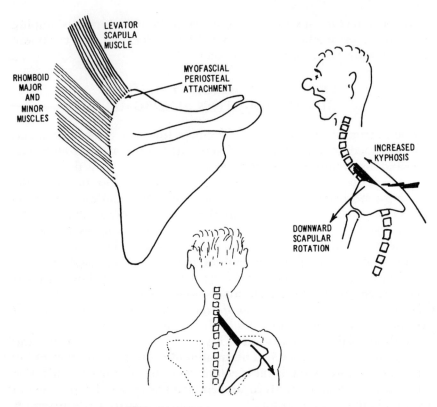

LEVATOR
SCAPULA
MUSCLE

MYOFASCIAL
PERIOSTEAL
ATTACHMENT

RHOMBOID
MAJOR
AND
MINOR
MUSCLES

INCREASED
KYPHOSIS

DOWNWARD
SCAPULAR
ROTATION

FIGURE 105. Scapulocostal syndrome. Pain located by the patient in the upper inter-scapular area and surmised to be between the medial border of the shoulder blade and the underlying rib cage, is a *myofascio-periostitis*. The "trigger area" is the site of attachment of the levator scapula muscle to the upper medial angle of the scapula. The mechanism is postural and tension traction of the attachment site.

drugs such as Butazolidin, brief steroid therapy, local procaine infil-tration into the trigger area, and posture training. In making this diag-nosis, one must always remain aware of the possible referred pain from heart or pulmonary disease.

FIBROMYOSITIS

Fibromyositis has long been considered by many to be a specific disease entity that persists in tissues after trauma. Fibromyositis is manifested clinically by the findings of painful muscles, nodules, stiffness, and spasm. This pathological syndrome is considered by many to be the most common cause of musculoskeletal pain but its existence is completely denied by others.[8, 9]

This condition has been designated as fibrositis, fibromyositis, myofascitis, interstitial myofasciitis, tension myositis, psychogenic rheumatism, and numerous other terms.

The subjective criteria for the "fibrositis syndrome" have been classified as:[10]

1. Aching and stiffness of more than three months' duration.
2. Morning aching and stiffness.
3. Aggravation of aching and stiffness by inclement weather.
4. Temporary relief by heat application.
5. Sleep disturbance of three or more months' duration.
6. Poor appetite.
7. Chronic fatigue and poor work tolerance for more than three months.

As many of these subjective symptoms are closely associated with psychological maladjustment, it is understandable that fibrositis has been considered to be a musculoskeletal manifestation of psychological problems.[11, 12]

Fibrositis has been defined as:[13]

A nonspecific inflammation of muscles, ligaments, muscle sheaths, fascial tissues, and aponeuroses and even the fibrous sheath of the nerves. The condition manifests itself as follows:
1. There is spontaneous, vague, poorly localized pain over the muscles involved—probably the muscles of the back, neck, and shoulders.
2. There is definite tenderness of the muscles to touch and pressure.
3. There is the same response to weather changes as is found in the joints in rheumatoid arthritis.
4. The condition responds in a similar manner as rheumatoid arthritis to therapeutic measures of rest, physiotherapy, immobilization, and antirheumatics.

Further complicating the specificity of the fibrositis syndrome is the fact that these patients have no fever, leukocytosis, increased sedimentation rate, altered serum enzyme levels, or any diagnostic electromyographic abnormalities.

Stimulation of a motor nerve, in a normal nerve-muscle unit causes release of acetylcholine in a very sharply demarcated area at the motor end plate. When there is denervation, there is a definite increase in the surface area of the muscle fiber that becomes sensitive to acetylcholine. This occurs within hours of denervation and becomes maximal within a

147

week.[20] Complete denervation is not necessary to cause muscle hypersensitivity. Minor degrees of trauma to the nerve can cause this resultant muscle fiber hypersensitivity.

In the denervated muscle there occurs fibrillation: a spontaneous electrical activity which occurs with *no* nerve release of the normal transmitter agent. This hypersensitive muscle fiber now responds to other (foreign) stimuli—from other nerve roots, preglanglionic autonomic fibers or from sensory nerve impulses. Spontaneous activity (sensitization) is considered to occur similiarly from denervation of the sympathetic nerve supply to the muscle.

Peripheral nerve disease or trauma has also been shown to affect the internuncial neurones of the dorsal roots in the spinal cord. Because supersensitivity occurs in all denervation—somatic, sympathetic, and central—painful tissues can result following any denervation regardless of the cause be it trauma, irritation infection, injection, and so forth.[21]

The myalgic hyperalgesia so characteristic of myofibrositic nodules is not found in normal muscle tissue. The nociceptors within muscle are found deep in the tissue and have a high threshold of excitation. They do not respond to ischemia or stretch but merely to deep strong pressure (fibers $A\delta$). The C fibers of muscle also have high thresholds but these are excited by ischemia or stretch.

Localized myopathy (myofibrositic nodules or "trigger") can result from local tissue trauma but may also occur secondarily to denervation of that particular muscle. Tenderness thus becomes maximal at the neuromuscular "motor point." This is, incidentally, the site of most trigger sites or referred trigger zones.[22] This phenomenon also explains the occurrence of localized muscle tenderness of the muscles (myotome) noted in cervical root entrapment or trauma. The resultant hypersensitive area can become self-perpetuating as is claimed in trigger zone mapping. This phenomenon also explains why many cases of so-called bursitis (tendonitis at the shoulder, elbow, or wrist) are essentially referred tender zones from cervical root lesions.[23]

Trauma is usually cited as the cause of the fibrositis. This trauma may be of any type or intensity varying from direct injury, sprain, postural musculoskeletal stress, emotional tension, exposure to cold, or a combination of these. Minor repeated traumas, none individually being considered significant, also have been considered as causative.

Characteristic of the fibrositis syndrome is the presence of "trigger areas." These triggers are small circumscribed hypersensitive areas in muscles or their surrounding connective tissues. These nodule-like sites are termed "trigger" because, when they are irritated or stimulated, they often refer pain to a distant "target" area. The target-trigger relationship is consistent and predictable. Pain in the target area is reproducible.

Once a trigger zone is initiated, and then the precipitating factor(s) eliminated, the trigger and its target zone may persist. This pain cycle becomes chronic and repetitive. The initiating trauma may have become forgotten.

Posture is a common inciting cause of fibrositic syndrome of the upper thoracic spine. This "scapulocostal syndrome" is a frequent sequela of the cervical syndrome. This is a syndrome of a slumped, rounded upper back posture. This posture may be secondary to occupation, fatigue, aging, or habit, or may be the musculoskeletal manifestation of depression.

The pain from this posture is felt in the interscapular muscles that are stressed by position of the shoulder girdles. These muscles, the levator scapulae and the rhomboids, are stressed beyond their physiological elongation and so held for prolonged periods of time. They become painful and irritable.

By virtue of the increased dorsal kyphosis, there results a compensation cervical lordosis which causes intervertebral foraminal closure, nerve root compression, excessive stress upon the facet joints of the cervical spine, and all the painful manifestations of this posture described in earlier chapters (see Figs. 76 and 105).

There are numerous other common fibrositic syndromes that are well documented in the literature and will not be discussed here.[12, 14, 15]

The diagnosis of a myofascial syndrome is based upon finding a circumscribed tender area that, when irritated by pressure, produces local tenderness and/or a referred pain. The "trigger" and its "target" zone are of a consistent pattern. There usually is a "jump sign" elicited in which the patient reacts to the pressure with an abrupt withdrawal. Vasomotor changes are frequently found in the trigger area and persist after local irritation. Muscle "spasm" is also found locally or in the target area. This "spasm" is essentially nodularity of the underlying muscles with firmness and tenderness. Local injection of the nodule with a small amount of local anesthetic is considered diagnostic.

Once the trigger area is located and the referral zone identified, local injection of the trigger with an anesthetic agent will usually interrupt the painful cycle. Similar benefit can be attained by spraying the tender area with ethyl chloride or vasocoolant spray. Stretch of the underlying muscle after spraying enhances the efficacy of the treatment. Deep sustained digital pressure exerted upon the trigger area has also been claimed to be beneficial and currently enjoys the term

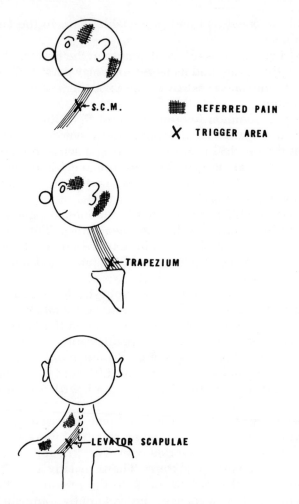

FIGURE 106. Trigger points and referred pain. Tender areas in various parts of the neck and shoulder, when irritated, can refer pain to distal sites.

"acupressure." Acupuncture of these trigger areas has also been described as beneficial.

The treatment is aimed at the eradication of the trigger area and not the referred zone (Fig. 106). To concentrate upon the latter frequently allows persistence of the syndrome after initial temporary relief.

PERICAPSULITIS SHOULDER PAIN

The "frozen shoulder" or the painful stiff shoulder[16] must be considered in differential diagnosis of neck-shoulder-arm pain, since it may be the sole cause of the pain or may be associated with and aggravating to the painful neck syndrome.

The most common cause of a painful restricted shoulder is tendonitis of the supraspinatous tendon. The tendon inevitably degenerates in the aging process due to the dependency of the arm and the numerous daily physical stresses placed on the arm and shoulder in everyday life. The tendon becomes constricted between the greater tuberosity of the humerus and the undersurface of the acromial process (Fig. 107). The inflamed tendon may go through the various stages of degeneration to ultimate calcification, but pain and restricted movement can occur at any stage. "Bursitis" of the shoulder, subacromial bursitis, is considered to be secondary to the tendonitis and rarely a single primary disease entity. The *bicipital tendonitis,* by its close anatomical relationship to the rotator cuff, is usually a concomitant lesion to rotator cuff inflammation. The bicipital syndrome, however, does exist as a specific entity in which the tendon may rupture or slip out of the bicipital groove, but this is very uncommon.

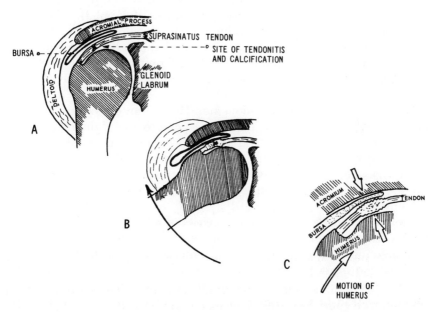

FIGURE 107. Glenohumeral movement. *A,* Normal relationship of the humerus in the glenoid fossa under the overhang of the acromial process. The supraspinatus tendon runs in this groove and is protected by the subacromial, subdeltoid bursa. In normal movement, the humeral head depresses as it abducts, and the tendon and the bursa move freely. *B* and *C,* The tendon is frayed, inflamed, or even calcified; thus, it is "pinched" between the humerus and the acromial process in arm abduction. Acute tendonitis and secondary bursitis result.

The history of acute tendonitis is an acute or an insidious pain in the shoulder region. The patient frequently localizes the pain in the upper lateral aspect of the arm in the region of the deltoid muscle insertion. Pain is frequent at night and is aggravated by abduction and external or internal rotation of the arm. "Combing the hair, reaching into the back pants pocket, reaching behind to fasten a bra," are movements that elicit pain early in the condition. If the condition progresses, the shoulder becomes "frozen" so that no movement is possible.

The clinical diagnosis is most characteristically made by observing the "shrugging" of the shoulder when the patient attempts side abduction of the arm. This shrug occurs because the *scapulo-humeral rhythm* is impaired. Normally, as the arm abducts, a synchronous rotation of the scapula accompanies the glenohumeral abduction. For every 10 degrees of glenohumeral abduction, there are 5 degrees of scapular rotation, a 2:1 ratio. If the glenohumeral movement is impaired, the scapula rotates fully with no arm abduction; thus the *shoulder shrugs* (Fig. 108).

The physician can observe impaired movement and pain by having the patient actively (or the physician passively) put the shoulder through the range of motion: abduction, overhead elevation, external rotation, and internal rotation (placing the hand behind the back and reaching between the shoulder blades). Comparing these with the "normal" side as well as observing which movements produce pain is informative.

Observing crepitation on movement is of limited value. Tenderness, if present, is felt at the bicipital groove region of the rotator cuff and is often too deep and too vague to be more than an "added" finding. X-ray revelation of calcification per se does *not* make the diagnosis since calcium may be seen in painless shoulders, and painful shoulders are most frequently seen with no X-ray evidence of calcium.

Treatment of the acute phase consists of a *brief* period of support with a sling and relief of pain by oral antiphlogistic drugs, ice packs, and injection of Novocaine and cortisone into the region of the rotator cuff and the supraspinatus tendon. All of these early measures are to relieve pain and decrease inflammation within a small area that could ultimately lead to a frozen shoulder. Pendular exercises of the arm should be started within the first few days.

As the acute phase subsides, the treatment includes a full range of motion exercise of the shoulder, application of heat, and improvement of posture. Surgery to disperse or remove the calcium is occasionally necessary when conservative measures fail. Surgery may include

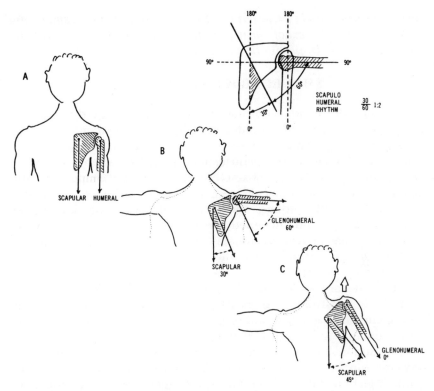

FIGURE 108. Scapulohumeral rhythm of shoulder movement. *A*, Loose-hanging arm with the scapula and humerus at 0°. *B*, Normal abduction during which, for every 15° of total abduction, 10° occur at the glenohumeral joint and 5° due to rotation of the scapula. *C*, When obstruction exists at the glenohumeral joint, the scapular movement exceeds or is the only movement of the shoulder girdle, and "shrugging" occurs.

open removal of the calcium deposit, manipulation, or needling and irrigation.

Since the *shrugging mechanism* uses the neck muscles, including the scalenes, and the neck is frequently held in spasm as a protective action, the symptoms of the anticus scalene syndrome may be mimicked. The neck symptoms of cervical diskogenic disease may also be aggravated. Determining the cause of the pain and verifying that the shoulder glenohumeral impairment is at fault requires careful evaluation. The shoulder site is indicated by the neck having a good range of motion and not reproducing the pain by its movement, pain being elicited by shoulder movement, "shrugging" on attempting abduction of the shoulder and arm, usually no distal subjective symptoms of paresthesia, and a negative neurological examination.

Again, *by reproducing the pain with a position or a movement and understanding the exact nature of that position or movement, the mechanism of pain production is understood.*

SHOULDER-HAND SYNDROME

The shoulder-hand syndrome,[17] also called reflex dystrophy or causalgia,[18] is a painful shoulder with limited movement *and* symptoms of swelling, pain, stiffness, sweating, and color changes of the hand. The changes in the hand usually progress in three stages: (1) local pain of a "burning" characteristic, vasomotor changes of coldness and perspiration or a cold, red, moist hand, stiffness, and superficial sensitivity, (2) coldness and stiffness in which the skin appears white, creaseless, and thickened, the joints actively and passively lose range, and muscle atrophy appears, and (3) the hand pale and thin, marked muscular atrophy, and the joints contracted. Osteoporosis is seen early on X-rays.

The causes of shoulder-hand syndrome[19] may be myocardial, posthemiplegic, posttraumatic, postherpetic, or secondary to cervical diskogenic disease and shoulder pericapsulitis. Many times the exact cause remains unknown. Treatment consists of encouraged, *if not forced,* motion of the hand and shoulder *in spite of pain,* sympathetic procaine blocks, paraffin baths to the hands, and procaine and cortisone injections into the shoulder and trigger points. Occasionally, it may even be necessary to perform sympathectomy.

The mechanism is postulated to be a reflex of pain sensations through sensory nerve roots and their sympathetic nerves to an internuncial pool in the spinal cord. The circuit is that of initiation by distal pain and sympathetic transmission to cause vasomotor action by reflex action (see Fig. 35B).

In later stages the diagnosis is evident. It is in the early stages, when the shoulder is "stiff" and the hand has vague symptoms of pain and paresthesia, that the diagnosis is most difficult and must be differentiated from other neck, nerve root irritation, shoulder pericapsulitis, and related conditions.

CARPAL TUNNEL SYNDROME

Symptoms felt in the hand from median nerve compression at the wrist will mimic nerve root compression at the cervical intervertebral foramina, symptoms of the anterior scalene neurovascular bundle compression, and even early hand-shoulder syndrome signs.

The cardinal symptoms of this disorder are paresthesia and pain referred to the fingers and hand in the distribution of the median nerve, numbness of the fingers, muscular weakness, clumsiness, and some trophic changes in the fingers. The paresthesia is described as tingling "pins and needles" that awaken the patient during the night. The pain is a "burning" sensation, and the weakness manifests itself as "clumsiness," "dropping things," and so forth. The symptoms refer mostly to the middle and index fingers and, to a lesser degree, the thumb. The little finger, not being innervated by the median nerve, is spared (Fig. 109).

The findings are those of impaired pin prick sensation in the palmar aspects of the terminal phalanges of the involved fingers. Loss of light

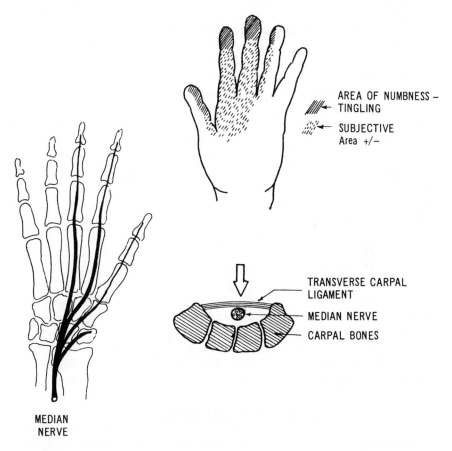

AREA OF NUMBNESS – TINGLING

SUBJECTIVE Area +/−

TRANSVERSE CARPAL LIGAMENT

MEDIAN NERVE

CARPAL BONES

MEDIAN NERVE

FIGURE 109. Carpal tunnel syndrome. Paresthesia and anesthesia occur from compression of the median nerve or its circulation at the carpal row of bone distal to the wrist. The compression occurs between the carpal bones and the transverse carpal ligament. The sensory distribution is depicted. Of clinical significance is the absence of subjective and objective dysesthesia of the little finger. Compression of the compartment is clinically reduplicated by a sustained flexion of the hand upon the forearm.

touch, vibration sense, and thermal appreciation is unusual. Motor weakness of the abductor and opponens of the thumb is difficult to ascertain unless marked and accompanied by atrophy.

A valuable test is to *reproduce the symptoms* by holding the wrist firmly and fully flexed upon the forearm for several minutes. A similar test to compress the circulation and reduplicate the symptoms is advocated by means of the pressure cuff, but this test has usually been unsatisfactory. The "Tinel sign" (reproducing tingling by percussion of the median nerve at the wrist) is disappointingly infrequent in spite of the claims made in the literature. X-rays may reveal bony changes at the wrist, but the syndrome is basically the history and reproduction of symptoms as described.

Treatment is either conservative, by immobilization of the wrist in a plaster cast, or surgical release of the transverse carpal ligament (flexor retinaculum). The conservative approach of resting the wrist in a neutral position for two weeks may in some patients result in permanent cure. If relief is afforded but is transient, it has the benefit of establishing the diagnosis, and the recurrence can be cured by surgery. Using night splints only, injecting the tunnel with cortisone, or using modalities such as ultrasound have been ineffective.

The EMG is very valuable in diagnosis, providing the motor portion of the nerve has been sufficiently compressed long enough to cause demyelinization. Numbness and tingling may become prolonged or permanent before the EMG is positive. Conduction time EMG studies are now available that reveal a nerve compression deficit, but this test is still unavailable in many clinics.

BRACHIAL PLEXUS NEURITIS (PLEXITIS)

This disease is relatively infrequent, but it must be considered in shoulder, arm, and hand pain. The onset is acute and usually consists of excruciating pain in the shoulder and down the arm. Weakness of the arm and hand is frequent, early, and may involve any or all of the peripheral nerves. Numbness is also usual. Because the inflammation is at the plexus level, the manifestation is of any or all of the roots of the plexus. The condition used to be a result of serum injections; but since serum is now rarely used, most etiologies are unknown.

A sling to support the arm and relieve traction on the plexus, medication for relief of pain, and strengthening of the weak muscles once the pain has subsided are the most that can be offered as treatment.

SUMMARY

Many conditions will simulate the symptoms and resemble the findings of cervical diskogenic pain, both locally in the neck and in its referred aspect. Confirming the source of trouble in the neck, under-standing the mechanism by which the symptoms are caused, and rec-ognizing the tissues capable of eliciting these signs are of utmost importance. A careful, meaningful history and physical examination usually reveal the problem clearly. A diagnosis need not be a diag-nosis by exclusion. The cause may remain unknown, but not the pathomechanics. When the physician recognizes which symptoms can be reproduced and which movements and positions reproduce them, he should have no question as to diagnosis and proper treatment.

REFERENCES

1. Haymaker, W. and Woodhall, B.: Peripheral Nerve Injuries, 2d ed. Philadelphia, W. B. Saunders, 1953.
2. Urschel, H. C., et al.: Objective diagnosis (ulnar nerve conduction velocity) and current therapy of the thoracic outlet syndrome. Ann. Thorac. Surg. 12:608–20, 1971.
3. Gage, M. and Parnell, H.: Scalenus anticus syndrome. Am. J. Surg. 73:252–68, 1947.
4. Love, J. G.: Intractable pain in the neck and upper extremities with particular reference to protrusion of cervical disks. N. Carolina Med. J. 12:274–86, 1951.
5. Nachlas, I. W.: Scalenus anticus syndrome or cervical foraminal compression? South. Med. J. 35:663–7, 1942.
6. Falconer, M. A. and Weddel, G.: Costoclavicular compression of the subclavian artery and vein: Relation to scalenus anticus syndrome. Lancet 2:539–43, 1943.
7. Michele, A. A., et al.: Scapulocostal syndrome (fatigue-postural paradox). N.Y. State J. Med. 50:1353–6, 1950.
8. Travel, J. and Rinzler, S. H.: The myofascial genesis of pain. Postgrad. Med. 11:425–34, 1952.
9. Simons, D. G.: Muscle pain syndrome. Am. J. Phys. Med. 54:289–311, 1976.
10. Moldofsky, H., et al.: Musculoskeletal symptoms and non-R.E.M. sleep disturbance in patients with "fibrositis syndrome" and healthy subjects. Psychosom. Med. 37:341–51, 1975.
11. Tegner, W., O'Neill, D., and Kaldegg, A.: Psychogenic rheumatism. Br. Med. J. 2:201–4, 1949.
12. Smythe, H. H. and Moldofsky, H.: Two contributions to understanding of the "fi-brositis syndrome." Bull. Rheum. Dis. 28:828–931, 1977.
13. Steindler, A.: Lectures on the Interpretation of Pain in Orthopedic Practice. Charles C Thomas, Springfield, Ill., 1959.
14. Sola, A. E. and Kuitert, J. H.: Myofascial trigger-point pain in the neck and shoulder girdle: 100 cases treated by normal saline. Northwest Med. 54:980–4, 1955.
15. Bonica, J. J.: Management of myofascial pain syndrome in general practice. J.A.M.A. 133:732–8, 1957.
16. Bloch, J. and Fischer, F. K.: Probleme der Schulterfteife. Acta Rheumatol. 2 Documenta Geigy, 1958.
17. Graham, W. and Rosen, P.: The shoulder-hand syndrome. Bull. Rheum. Dis. 12:277–8, 1962.
18. Threadgill, F. D.: Causalgia. Bull. Georgetown Univ. Med. Cent. 2:110–2, 1948.
19. Molberg, E.: Shoulder-hand-finger syndrome. Surg. Clinic N. Am. 40:367–73, 1960.
20. Cannon, W. B. and Rosenblueth, A.: The Supersensitivity of Denervated Structures. New York, Macmillan, 1949, pp. 1–22, 185.
21. Gunn, C. C.: "Prespondylosis" and some pain syndromes following denervation supersensitivity. Spine 5:185–92, 1980.

22. Kraus, H.: Triggerpoints. N.Y. State J. Med. 73:1310–14, 1973.
23. Gunn, C. C. and Milbrandt, W. E.: Tenderness at motor points—an aid in the diagnosis of pain in the shoulder referred from the cervical spine. J.A.O.A. 77:196/ 75–212/91, 1977.

BIBLIOGRAPHY

Berge, P. V.: Myofascial pain syndromes. Postgrad. Med. 53:161–8, 1973.

Forster, F. M. and Kiesel, J. A.: Brachial plexus neuritis. Bull. Georgetown Univ. Med. Cent. 5:74–6, 1951.

Johnson, E. W., Wells, R. M., and Duran, R. J.: Diagnosis of carpal tunnel syndrome. Arch. Phys. Med. Rehabil. 43:414–9, 1962.

Kraft, G. H., Johnson, E. W., and LaBan, M. D.: The fibrositic syndrome. Arch. Phys. Med. Rehabil. 49:155–62, 1968.

Kraus, H.: Use of surface anesthesia in treatment of painful motion. J.A.M.A. 116:2582–3, 1941.

Index

ACCELERATION injury of neck, 73–93
Acute central spinal cord injury, 90–92
Adson test, 140
Anatomy. *See* Functional anatomy.
Annulus, 2
Anterior scalene syndrome, 139–143
Anxiety resulting from cervical injury, 134
Atlanto-axial joint, 20
Atlanto-epistrophic joint, 14
Atlas, 11, 14, 20, 28, 39
Axis, 14, 28, 39

BLOOD supply. *See* Vascular supply.
Brachial plexus neuritis, 156
Brachioradialis reflex, 67–68

CAPITAL extensors, 22–23
Capital flexors, 22–23
Carpal tunnel syndrome, 154–156
Center of gravity, 9
Cervical. *See also*, entries under Neck.
Cervical disk, 1–4
  disease of, 56–71
    degenerative, 94–105
    herniation, 58, 62–64, 96
    localization of root level in, 64–71
    radicular pain in, nature and mechanism of, 56–62
  pain and, 23–25, 62–64
Cervical nerves, 27–34, 39
  localization of pain and, 64–71
Cervical spine
  dislocation of, 85–86
  functional anatomy of, 1
    cervical nerves, 27–34

functional unit, 1–7
kinetic spine, 11–18
ligamentous support, 18–21
musculature of neck, 21–23
posture, 9–11
static spine, 8–9
sympathetic nervous system, 34–38
tissue sites of pain production, 23–27
upper cervical segments, 38
movement of, 11–18
physical examination of, 51
osteophyte formation in, 96–105
spondylosis of, 97–105
sprain of, 73–93
treatment of disorders of, 118–135
whiplash syndrome of, 73–93
Cervical spondylotic myelopathy, 106–110
  examination in, 112
  laboratory findings in, 112–113
  myelography in, 113–115
  prognosis in, 112
  symptoms of, 111
  treatment of, 115–116
Cervical vertebrae, 1–7
  movement and, 11–18
Claviculocostal syndrome, 143–145
Collar, cervical, in treatment of neck pain, 119–123
Compression-avulsion theory of whiplash injury, 80–82
Compression-plus-torque theory of whiplash injury, 82–84
Compression syndromes, 137–157
Contraction of muscle, pain and, 42–44

159

Cramps, 44
CSM. *See* Cervical spondylotic myelopathy.
Curves of spine, 8–10

DECELERATION injury of neck, 73–93
Degenerative disease of cervical disk, 94–105
Diagnosis
  differential, 137–139
  of anterior scalene syndrome, 139–143
  of brachial plexus neuritis, 156
  of carpal tunnel syndrome, 154–156
  of claviculocostal syndrome, 143–145
  of deceleration sprain injury, 92–93
  of fibromyositis, 146–150
  of neck pain, 50–55
  of pectoralis minor syndrome, 145
  of pericapsulitis shoulder pain, 150–154
  of scapulocostal syndrome, 145–146
  of shoulder-hand syndrome, 154
Disability, cervical disk disease, and, 56–71
Diseases of cervical disk, 56–71
  degenerative, 94–105
Dislocations of cervical spine, 52–53, 85–86
Disk, cervical, 1–4
  disease of, 56–71
    degenerative, 94–105
  herniation of, 62–64, 96
  intradiskal pressure, 2–3
  pain and, 23–25, 62–64
Diskography, 53–54, 57
Dural sleeve, 26

ELASTICITY of intervertebral disk, 3
Electromyography, 54–55
  in diagnosis of carpal tunnel syndrome, 156
Epineural sheath, 34
Examination in diagnosis of neck pain
  physical, 51–52
  X-ray, 52–55
Exercises in treatment of neck pain, 132
Extension, 14–18
  in physical examination of neck, 51

FATIGUE, posture and, 10–11
Fibromyositis, 146–150
Flexion, 14–18
  in physical examination of neck, 51

Fractures of cervical spine, 52–53
"Frozen shoulder," 150–154
Functional anatomy of cervical spine, 1
  cervical nerves, 27–34
  functional unit, 1–7
    degenerative changes in, 97–98
  kinetic spine, 11–18
  ligamentous support, 18–21
  musculature of neck, 21–23
  posture, 9–11
  static spine, 8–9
  sympathetic nervous system, 34–38
  tissue sites of pain production, 23–27
  upper cervical segments, 38
Fusion in treatment of cervical injury, 135

GLENOHUMERAL movement, 151
Gravity, center of, 8–9

HABIT, posture and, 11
Hard disk herniation, 64, 96
Headaches, tension, 42
Heat, in treatment of neck pain, 123–124
Hereditary influences on posture, 10
Herniation of cervical disk, 58, 62–64, 96
Hyperabduction syndrome, 145
Hyperextension injury
  acute central spinal cord injury, 90–92
  whiplash syndrome, 74–90
Hyperflexion injury
  acute central spinal cord injury, 90–92
  whiplash syndrome, 74–90

ICE packs, in treatment of neck pain, 124
Immobilization, in treatment of neck pain, 120–121, 124–125
Intradiskal pressure, 2–3
  degeneration of disk and, 95–96
Intervertebral disk, 1–4
Ischemia of muscle, pain and, 26–27, 43–44
Isometric contraction, 43
Isotonic contraction, 43

JOINT(S)
  atlanto-axial, 20
  atlanto-epistrophic, 14
  glenohumeral, 151
  of von Luschka, 7, 32, 96
  zygapophyseal, 32

KINETIC spine, 11–18

Kinetic spine—*continued*
  physical examination of, 51

LORDOSIS, 8–10
Ligamentous support of neck, 18–21
Localization of root level in cervical disk
    disease, 64–71
Lumbar spine, 5–8

MASSAGE, in treatment of neck pain, 124
Medication, in treatment of neck pain, 119
Movements of neck, 11–18
  physical examination of, 51
Musculature of neck, 21–23
  pain and, 26–27, 42–44
  response of, to whiplash, 77
Myalgia, 59
Myelography, 53, 113–115
Myelopathy, cervical spondylotic, 106–
    116
Myositis, 43

NECK. *See also,* entries under Cervical.
  dislocation of, 85–86
  disk disease in, 56–71
    degenerative, 94–105
  ligamentous support of, 18–21
  movements of, 11–18
    physical examination of, 51
  musculature of, 21–23
  pain in, 23–27
    diagnosis of, 50–55, 137–157
    originating in soft tissues, 42–48
  sprain of, 74–93
  sympathetic nervous system and, 34–38
  treatment of disorders of, 118–135
  whiplash syndrome of, 73–93
Nerves, cervical, 27–34, 39
  localization of pain and, 64–71
Neuralgia, 58
Nucleus pulposus, 2

OSTEOARTHRITIS, 44–46
Osteophytes, 96–105

PAIN
  in neck, 23–27
    diagnosis of, 50–55, 137–157
    disk disease and, 56–71
    originating in soft tissues, 42–48
    treatment of, 118–135
    whiplash and, 86

radicular, nature and mechanism of,
    56–62
  referred, 59, 65–71
Pectoralis minor syndrome, 145
Pericapsulitis shoulder pain, 150–154
Periradicular sheath, 34
Physical examination
  in cervical spondylotic myelopathy, 112
  in diagnosis of neck pain, 51–52
Pillow, cervical, in treatment of neck pain,
    123
Plexitis, 156
Posterior interspinous ligaments, 21
Posture, 9–11
  degenerative disk changes and, 102
Pronator reflex, 68

RADICULAR pain, nature and mechanism of,
    56–62
Referred pain, 59, 65–71
  in whiplash injury, 86
Reflex(es)
  brachioradialis, 67–68
  pronator, 68
Root level localization in cervical disk dis-
    ease, 64–71
Root pain, 60–61

SCAPULOCOSTAL syndrome, 145–146
Shoulder-hand syndrome, 154
Soft disk herniation, 64, 96
Soft tissues, neck pain originating in,
    42–48
Spine
  cervical
    dislocation of, 85–86
    functional anatomy of, 1
      cervical nerves, 27–34
      functional unit, 1–7
      kinetic spine, 11–18
      ligamentous support, 18–21
      musculature of neck, 21–23
      posture, 9–11
      static spine, 8–9
      sympathetic nervous system, 34–38
      tissue sites of pain production, 23–
          27
      upper cervical segments, 38
    movement and, 11–18
      physical examination of, 51
    osteophyte formation in, 96–105
    spondylosis of, 97–116

Spine—*continued*
    sprain of, 73–93
      treatment of disorders of, 118–135
      whiplash syndrome of, 73–93
    lumbar, 1, 5–7
Spondylosis, 97–105
Spondylotic myelopathy, cervical, 106–116
Spondylotic radiculopathy, 60
Sprain, cervical, 74–93
    treatment of, 118–135
Static spine, 8–9
Sternal-occipital-mandibular immobilizer, 121
Surgery in treatment of cervical injury, 134–135
Subluxation(s)
    diagnosis of deceleration injury and, 92–93
    syndrome of central spinal cord injury, 90–92
    treatment of, 118–135
    whiplash syndrome, 73–90
Sympathetic chain, 36
Sympathetic nervous system, 34–38
    whiplash injury and, 86–90
Syndrome(s)
    anterior scalene, 139–143
    carpal tunnel, 154–156
    claviculocostal, 143–145
    compression, 137–157
    "frozen shoulder," 150–154
    hyperabduction, 145
    pectoralis minor, 145
    scapulocostal, 145–146
    shoulder-hand, 154
    whiplash, 73–93

TENDONITIS of shoulder, 152
Tension
    pain and, 42, 50–51
    posture and, 11
Tension myositis, 43

Tissues, soft, neck pain originating in, 42–48
Torticollis, 46–47
Traction, in treatment of neck pain, 124–131
Tranquilizers, in treatment of neck pain, 119
Transverse ligament, 20
Treatment, 118–135
    of anticus scalene syndrome, 141–143
    of brachial plexus neuritis, 156
    of carpal tunnel syndrome, 156
    of cervical spondylotic myelopathy, 115–116
    of claviculocostal syndrome, 144–145
    of fibromyositis, 149–150
    of pericapsulitis shoulder pain, 152–153
    of scapulocostal syndrome, 145–146

UPPER cervical segments, 38–39

VASCULAR supply to cervical disks, 4, 94
Vertebrae, cervical, 1–7
    movement and, 11–18
Vertebral nerve, 36, 37
Vertebral plexus, 37
Von Luschka, joints of, 7, 32, 96

WHIPLASH, 73–90
    diagnosis of deceleration injury and, 92–93
    neurologic symptoms of, 86–90
    syndrome of central spinal cord injury and, 90–92
    theories of mechanism of, 80–84

X-RAY examination
    in diagnosis of neck pain, 52–55
    in deceleration sprain injury, 92–93
    in cervical spondylotic myelopathy, 112–113

ZYGAPOPHYSEAL joints, 32